Mind Your Mind

Develop Self Care Mental Habits, Nurture and Cultivate Your Mind and increase your Intellectual Well-Being

Manjul Tewari

www.manjultewari.com

MASTER YOUR LIFE WITH THE MASTERY SERIES

Y OU CAN CHECK OUT the other books in the series , "Unleashing to Master the Power Within "below:

Scan below to learn about Ultimate Mindset Mastery Series

Scan this QR code to
learn about Ultimate Mindset
Mastery Series

Scan this QR Code to learn about Unleashing Mindset Mastery Series

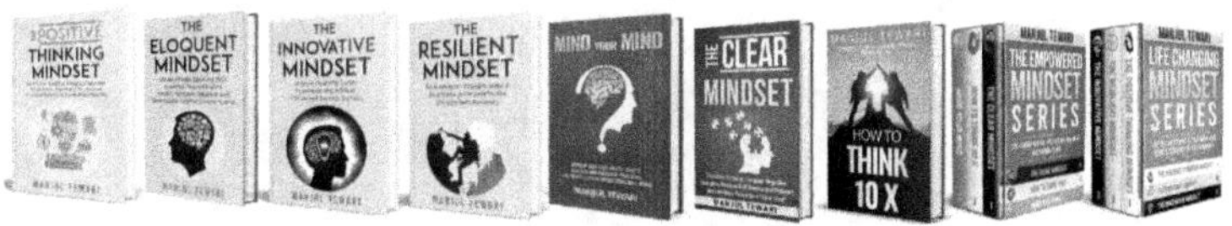

Mindset Mastery Series

YOUR FREE GIFT

As a token of my thanks for taking out time to read my book , I would like to offer you a gift.

Download your Free PDF eBook

<u>10 Useful Ways of Talking To Any Body</u>

clicking the link

https://www.manjultewari.com/my-free-e-book/

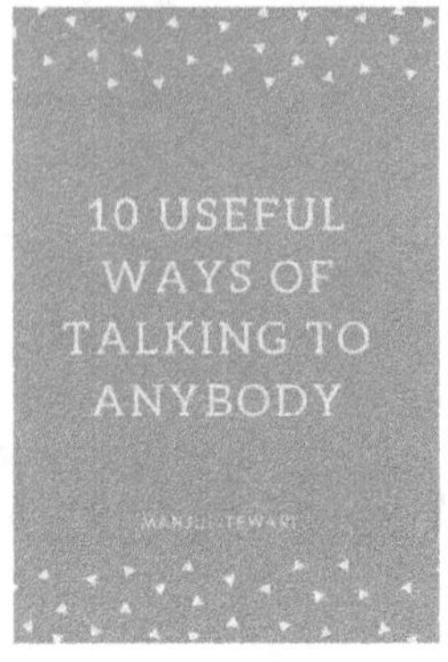

Ten Useful Ways of Talking To Anybody

OR

Scan this QR code to claim your free E Book.

*Scan this QR Code with your
smart phone and download your
free e book*

Published by **Mr. Manjul Tewari**
P-24, Engineer Park Apartment, Omega Sector-1
Greater Noida, UP, India 201308

Contents

CHAPTER ONE

INTRODUCTION

TECHNOLOGY IS A DOUBLE-EDGED sword, as it has the potential to both help and hinder us. Because of this, it is important that we remember the importance of going out of our way to stimulate our minds. Even though we are constantly bombarded with information, much of the content we encounter is seemingly pointless.

To stay focused and attentive towards what matters most, we need to find ways to actively engage in stimulating behaviours like reading, writing, and puzzle-solving. These activities can be very helpful in keeping our minds sharp. If you're looking for ways to improve your mental focus, then read on for some great tips!

Sitting down for long periods of time can reduce cognitive function, cause back and neck pain, and lead to weight gain. Make sure you get up and move around as often as possible, even if it's just for a few minutes at a time--you'll reap the mental and physical benefits!

Stimulation keeps our minds active and engaged, which has a number of benefits. For one, it can help stave off mental decline in old age. It can also improve our memory and cognitive function, help us learn new things more easily, and keep our thinking processes sharp. Additionally, stimulation can help alleviate boredom and make us feel more alert and awake.

All of these benefits are important for maintaining a high quality of life as we age. So, if you're looking for ways to keep your mind healthy and active, Stimulation is a great place to start!

It has long been said that we only use a small percentage of our brain power. Imagine what we could achieve if we could learn to tap into more of our mental potential! Here are some ways to stimulate your mind and unleash your hidden genius:

1. **Get physical exercise.** Exercise not only benefits our bodies but also our cognitive abilities. A recent study found that just 30 minutes of moderate aerobic exercise can immediately improve executive function and working memory.

2. **Make time for creative activities**. Give yourself time each day to do something creative, whether it's painting, writing, playing music, or gardening. According to research, engaging in creative pursuits can increase intelligence and help stave off age-related cognitive decline.

3. **Learn something new**. When you challenge your brain with new information, you create new neural connections that can improve cognitive function. So go ahead and sign up for that cooking class or start studying a new language!

4. **Get enough sleep**. Sleep is essential for both physical and mental health. A good night's sleep can help improve memory, concentration, and problem-solving skills.

5. **Eat a healthy diet**. Eating healthy foods helps protect the brain from damage and supports cognitive function. Be sure to include plenty of fresh fruits and vegetables and grains in your diet.

There are many ways to stimulate our minds, and it really depends on what we're looking for. If we want to learn something new, we might read a book or take a class.

If we want to relax and de-stress, we might do some yoga or meditation. And if we want to get creative, we might try painting or writing. Ultimately, it's up to us to decide what will work best for us at any given moment.

But if we're open to trying new things, the possibilities are endless. Self-care is a phrase often used in the well-being, wellness, and mental health communities. The goal of self-care is to improve your mental and physical well-being by taking time for yourself. In order to come up with your own list of self-care activities, take some time to reflect on what you enjoy doing.

Self-care has become a hot topic in recent years, with more people than ever increasingly looking for ways to take care of themselves and make their lives better. With that said, it's no surprise that mental self-care is one of the most popular topics out there.

The problem is figuring out how to actually do it. Let us take a look at writing is hard - it can take a lot of time and effort, and the payoff isn't always instantaneous. It's difficult to find the right type of routine to fit your needs as a writer: you might try waking up earlier so you have enough time to write, but end up feeling sleep-deprived. You might force yourself to go on daily walks in order to clear your mind, but then you have no energy for writing.

The struggle with maintaining self-care and mental habits is real! Let us look at some helpful tips on what you can do to start developing your own self-care mental habits! Practising self-care is much like practising a sport.

It needs to be practised often in order to condition your brain to perform well. Some people might feel that they don't have time (or the energy) to engage in self-care rituals every day, but it's important to at least take some time for yourself during the week!

Self-care is any activity that we do deliberately in order to take care of our mental, emotional, and physical health. Although it's often seen as something we do when we're feeling stressed or overwhelmed, self-care is actually preventive and proactive. By making self-care a regular part of our lives, we can avoid burnout and keep ourselves feeling our best.

There are many different types of self-care, but some common examples include exercise, eating healthy foods, getting enough sleep, spending time outdoors, taking breaks from work or other obligations, spending time with loved ones, practising meditation or relaxation techniques, and writing in a journal.

Everyone's needs are different, so it's important to find what works for you. Experiment and find what activities make you feel refreshed and recharged.

Making self-care a priority can be difficult, but it's worth it. When we take care of ourselves, we're better able to take care of others and meet the demands of our everyday lives. By taking the time to nurture our minds, body, and spirit, we can live happier and healthier lives.

Self-care is important because it helps you stay healthy both physically and mentally. When you take care of yourself, you're able to better manage stress and avoid burnout. Additionally, self-care can improve your mood and increase your overall sense of well-being.

There are many different ways to practice self-care, but some of the most common include exercises, getting enough sleep, eating a healthy diet, and spending time with loved ones. Everyone's needs are different, so it's important to find what works best for you. Ultimately, the goal is to find balance in your life and make time for activities that make you happy and help you relax.

There are many different self-care activities that people can do to help themselves feel better mentally and physically. Some common self-care activities include:

-eating healthy foods and getting enough exercise

-getting enough sleep and rest

-taking breaks when needed and relaxing

-connecting with friends, family, or others for support

-doing things that you enjoy or make you feel good

These are just a few examples of self-care activities, but there are many more out there. It is important to find what works best for you and to do what you can to take care of yourself.

Self-care is important for maintaining your physical and mental health. There are many ways to incorporate self-care into your daily routine.

Here are a few ideas:

1. **Make time for yourself every day.** Dedicate at least 30 minutes to an activity that you enjoy, such as reading, writing, hiking, biking, or taking a bath.

2. **Eat healthy meals and snacks**. Fuel your body with nutritious foods that will give you energy and help you feel your best.

3. **Get enough sleep.** Most people need 7-8 hours of sleep per night. Consider going to bed and waking up at the same time each day to help regulate your body's natural sleep rhythm.

4. **Take breaks throughout the day.** If you're feeling overwhelmed or stressed, take a few minutes to yourself to relax and rejuvenate. Take deep breaths, stretch, or meditate.

5. **Connect with loved ones.** Spending time with people who make you happy can reduce stress and promote positive emotions. Whether it's catching up with a friend over coffee or Facetiming with family members, social interactions can boost your mood and well-being.

Self-care is important for a variety of reasons. It can help reduce stress, improve your mood, and increase your overall sense of well-being. Additionally, a self-care routine can help you to be more productive and efficient in other areas of your life. When you take care of yourself, you are better able to take care of others.

A self-care routine does not need to be complicated or time-consuming. Something as simple as taking a few minutes each day to do something that you enjoy can make a big difference. Self-care is all about making choices that will lead to a healthier, happier you. So, experiment and find what works best for you!

Self-care is important for our physical, mental, and emotional well-being. It can be hard to find time for self-care when we are busy with work, family, and other obligations. Here are some tips for making time for self-care:

1. **Schedule time for yourself:** Set aside some time each day or week for activities that help you relax and rejuvenate. This could be something as simple as reading a book, taking a bath, going for a walk, or taking a yoga class.

2. **Make self-care a priority**: Don't let other things always take precedence over taking care of yourself. If you don't have time for a full self-care routine, do something small that will make a difference in how you feel.

3. **Find creative ways to incorporate self-care into your day:** If you can't find large chunks of time to devote to self-care, look for ways to sneak it into your day. Take a few minutes here and there to do something special for yourself. Listen to your favourite music while you cook dinner, take a break at work to read a few pages of your book, or squeeze in a quick workout during your lunch break.

4. **Ask for help**: If you're struggling to find time for self-care, ask others for help. Family and friends can pitch in with childcare or household duties so that you can have some extra time for yourself. You can also

Self-care is so important for our overall well-being, yet it's often something we forget to do. We hope this introduction has helped you understand what self-care is and why it's vital for a happy, healthy life. Remember to make time for yourself every day, even if it's just a few minutes. Your mind, body and soul will thank you for it!

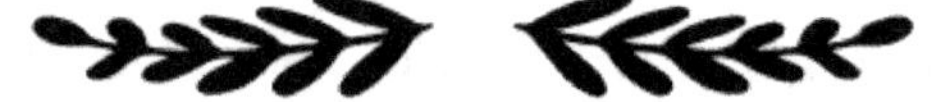

CHAPTER TWO

DEVELOP DAILY SELF CARE MENTAL HABITS

BEST RELAXATION TECHNIQUES

RELAXATION TECHNIQUES ARE A form of self-care that can help reduce stress, and anxiety, and promote overall well-being. There are many different relaxation techniques that can be used, and finding the right one for you may take some trial and error. We will explore some of the most popular relaxation techniques and offer tips on how to get started.

From deep breathing exercises to yoga and meditation, there are many ways to promote Relaxation. So, find what works best for you and start reaping the benefits today!

If you're like most people, chances are you don't make relaxation a priority. But what if I told you that relaxation is one of the keys to a happy and healthy life?

It's important to find what works best for you when it comes to relaxation techniques. We will explore some of the most popular relaxation techniques and offer tips on how to get started.

Relaxation techniques overview

There are many relaxation techniques that can be useful in managing stress and anxiety. Some common relaxation techniques include:

-Deep breathing: Deep breathing is a simple but effective relaxation technique that can be done anywhere. Simply take a deep breath in through your nose, filling your lungs as much as possible. Then slowly exhale through your mouth. Repeat this several times.

-Progressive muscle relaxation: This technique involves tensing and relaxing different muscle groups in the body, one at a time. Start by tensing the muscles in your toes for a few seconds, then relax them. Work your way up the body, tensing and relaxing muscles group by group until you reach your head and neck.

-**Visualization:** Visualization involves picturing a peaceful or calming scene in your mind. It can help to focus on specific details, such as the colours of the scene, the sounds you hear, or the sensations you feel.

-**Yoga: Yoga** combines physical activity with breathing exercises and relaxation techniques. There are many different types of yoga, so it's important to find one that's right for you.

-**Tai chi**: Tai chi is a Chinese martial art that involves slow, graceful movements and deep breathing. Like yoga, tai chi can help to reduce stress and improve overall health.

-**Meditation:** Meditation involves focusing your attention on a specific object, thought, or activity. It can help to clear your mind and improve your focus.

Relaxation techniques can be used on their own or as part of a larger stress management plan.

Breathing exercises

Breathing exercises are a great way to relax and de-stress. There are many different breathing exercises you can do, but some of the most effective ones are diaphragmatic breathing, progressive muscle relaxation, and controlled breathing.

Diaphragmatic breathing is a great way to reduce stress and promote relaxation. To do this exercise, sit in a comfortable position with your back straight and your shoulders relaxed. Place one hand on your stomach just below your belly button.

Slowly inhale through your nose, allowing your stomach to expand as you fill your lungs with air. As you exhale through your mouth, purse your lips and push all the air out of your lungs until your stomach contracts. Repeat this process for 10-15 minutes.

Controlled breathing is another simple but effective relaxation technique that can be done anywhere at any time. To do this exercise, simply breathe in through your nose for a count of four.

Breathe out through your mouth for a count of four. Repeat this process for 10-15 minutes.

Guided imagery

Guided imagery is a relaxation technique that involves using your imagination to create peaceful images in your mind. This exercise can be done anywhere at any time and is a great way to reduce stress and promote relaxation. To do this exercise, sit or lie down in a comfortable position and close your eyes.

Take a few deep breaths and focus on the image you want to create in your mind. It can be anything from a tranquil scene in nature to a calm, safe place. Once you have the image in your mind, focus on the details and try to make it as realistic as possible. Stay focused on the image for 5-10 minutes before opening your eyes and taking a few deep breaths.

Yoga

Yoga is a relaxation technique that can be used to ease the mind and body. Yoga poses, or asanas, are designed to stretch and tone the muscles, improve flexibility, and release tension.

Breath work, or pranayama, is an important part of yoga and helps to control the breath and calm the mind. Meditation is another important element of yoga practice and can be used to focus the mind and promote inner peace.

Inhale as you return to the starting position. Exhale as you repeat the movement on the other side. Continue moving slowly and smoothly through the movements, focusing on your breath and body posture.

Yoga is a great way to reduce stress, increase flexibility, and improve overall health. There are many different types of yoga, so there is sure to be one that is perfect for you. Some of the most popular types of yoga include:

Hatha Yoga: This type of yoga focuses on physical postures and breathing exercises. It is a great way to reduce stress and tension in the body.

Bikram Yoga: Also known as "hot yoga", this type of yoga is done in a heated room to help loosen muscles and promote detoxification.

Vinyasa Yoga: This type of yoga focuses on continuous, flowing movements. It is a great workout and can also help reduce stress.

There are many other types of yoga, so be sure to explore until you find the perfect one for you.

Mindfulness meditation

Mindfulness meditation is a great way to focus on the present moment and let go of stress and anxiety. To do this exercise, find a comfortable place to sit or lie down. Close your eyes and take a few deep breaths. Focus on your breath and the sensations in your body. If your mind starts to wander, simply bring your attention back to your breath. Continue this process for 10-15 minutes.

Progressive muscle relaxation

Progressive muscle relaxation is another excellent way to reduce stress and promote relaxation. This exercise involves tensing and relaxing different muscle groups in the body. Start by tensing the muscles in your feet and ankles for 5-10 seconds before relaxing them completely.

Then move up to your calves, thighs, hips, hands, arms, neck, and face, and tense each group of muscles for 5-10 seconds before relaxing them completely.

Once you've gone through all the muscle groups, take a few deep breaths and feel the tension leaving your body. Progressive muscle relaxation is a technique that can be used to relieve stress and tension. It involves the systematic tensing and relaxing of different muscle groups in the body.

This process can help to improve circulation, increase the range of motion, and reduce pain. It can also be used as a way to prepare for or recover from strenuous activity.

To do progressive muscle relaxation, start by sitting or lying in a comfortable position. Take a deep breath in and then exhale slowly. As you exhale, tense the muscles in your toes for 10 seconds. Then relax the muscles for 10 seconds as you breathe out.

Continue this pattern working your way up through each muscle group in your body: feet, calves, thighs, hips, abdomen, chest, arms, hands, neck, jaw, and face. Make sure to spend an equal amount of time tensing and relaxing each muscle group.

Visualization

There are a number of different visualization techniques that can be used for relaxation. One popular technique is to imagine a peaceful or calming scene, such as a beach or a forest. Other techniques include focusing on your breath and counting each inhale and exhale or picturing a relaxing colour or image.

Visualization can be used anywhere and at any time – you don't need any special equipment or environment. Simply close your eyes and focus on the image, scene or sensation you want to create in your mind. The more vivid and realistic you can make it, the more effective it will be.

Regular practice of visualization can help to reduce stress levels, improve sleep quality and increase overall feelings of well-being.

Aromatherapy

Aromatherapy is a form of alternative medicine that uses essential oils to promote relaxation and well-being. Aromatherapy can be used in a variety of ways, including inhalation and topical application.

The most popular essential oils used in aromatherapy include lavender, chamomile, and peppermint. These oils are believed to have properties that can help to relieve stress, anxiety, and tension. Aromatherapy is often used as a complementary treatment to other relaxation techniques, such as yoga or meditation.

Tai chi

Tai chi is a Chinese martial art that involves slow, graceful movements and deep breathing. Tai chi can be done alone or in a group, and there is no need for any special equipment or clothing.

Regular practice of tai chi can help to reduce stress, improve balance and coordination, and increase flexibility and range of motion. Tai chi can also be used as a form of self-defence.

To do tai chi, start by standing with your feet shoulder-width apart and your arms at your sides. Slowly shift your weight to your left foot and raise your right hand in front of you, keeping your palm open. As you exhale, turn your palm to face downwards and sweep your hand down to your left side.

Tai chi is a form of martial arts that originated in China. It is based on the principle of using slow, controlled movements to achieve balance and harmony between the body and mind. Tai chi is often described as "meditation in motion" because it promotes relaxation and stress relief.

There are many benefits of practising tai chi, including improved balance and coordination, reduced stress and anxiety, better sleep, and increased strength and flexibility. Tai chi can be done by people of all ages and fitness levels. It is a safe, low-impact form of exercise that can be done indoors or outdoors.

If you're looking for a way to relax and de-stress, tai chi may be a good option for you.

Meditation

Meditation is a popular relaxation technique that can be used to help reduce stress, anxiety, and tension. There are many different ways to meditate, so it's important to find a method that works best for you. One of the most common ways to meditate is to focus on your breath. Sit or lie down in a comfortable position and close your eyes.

Slowly inhale and exhale, paying attention to your breath as it enters and leaves your body. If your mind starts to wander, simply redirect your focus back to your breath. You can also try focusing on a mantra or word that you repeat to yourself during meditation.

Spending even a few minutes meditating can help to calm and focus the mind. With regular practice, meditation can help to reduce stress levels, improve sleep quality, and increase overall well-being.

Tips for choosing the right relaxation technique

There is no one-size-fits-all answer to this question, as the best relaxation technique for you may vary depending on your individual needs and preferences. However, there are a few key things to keep in mind when choosing a relaxation technique that will help you find the one that works best for you.

First, consider what you want to achieve through relaxation. Do you want to reduce stress, improve sleep, or boost your mood? Once you know what your goal is, you can narrow down your options and choose a technique that is best suited to help you achieve it.

Second, think about what type of environment you feel most relaxed in. Do you prefer being outdoors in nature, or indoors in a quiet room? This will help guide you towards techniques that will be most effective for you.

Finally, consider your personal preferences and needs when choosing a relaxation technique. For example, if you have trouble sitting still, then a moving meditation like Tai Chi or Yoga might be a better option for you than something like mindfulness meditation. Trust your instincts and go with what feels right for you.

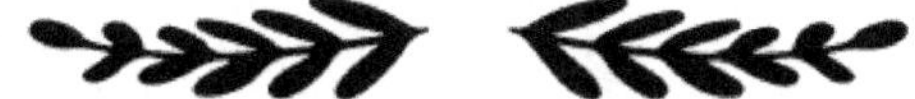

CHAPTER THREE

DEVELOP INTELLECTUAL WELL BEING

WHAT IS INTELLECTUAL WELL-BEING?

"Intellectual growth should commence at birth and cease only at death"-

Intellectual well-being is a state of being in which a person's intellectual needs are met and they are able to think critically and creatively. A person with intellectual well-being is curious and open-minded and has a growth mindset. They are also able to manage their emotions, set and achieve goals, and deal with stress in healthy ways.

Intellectual well-being is the state of being intellectually healthy. It is characterized by a love of learning, critical thinking skills, and a willingness to engage in intellectual pursuits. Intellectual well-being is important for both individuals and society as a whole.

Individuals who are intellectually well are able to think critically and solve problems. They are also more likely to be engaged in their communities and contribute to the common good. In addition, people who are intellectually well tend to be happier and more fulfilled than those who are not.

There are many ways to develop intellectual well-being. One way is to engage in lifelong learning. This can be done by taking classes, attending lectures, and reading books. Another way to develop intellectual well-being is to participate in activities that require critical thinking, such as debates, discussion groups, and puzzles. Finally, it is also important to spend time with people who value intellect and share your interests.

How to develop intellectual well being

We all know the importance of physical well-being, but what about intellectual well-being? Just as our bodies need exercise and proper nutrition to function at their best, our minds need stimulation and challenges to stay sharp. Unfortunately, in today's society, it's easy to get caught up in the hustle and bustle of everyday life and neglect our intellectual well-being.

If you're looking to improve your mental health and cognitive function, here are some tips on how to develop intellectual well-being. However, it's important to remember that your mental health is just as important as your physical health

There are many different ways to develop intellectual well-being. However, some things are more important than others. Here are a few tips on how to develop intellectual well-being:

1. **Read regularly**. Reading stimulates the mind and helps you learn new things. It can also help you become more critical and analytical.

2. **Write regularly.** Writing is a great way to organize your thoughts and express yourself clearly. It can also help you improve your communication skills.

3. **Be curious**. Curiosity is the key to learning new things and expanding your knowledge base. Never stop asking questions and seeking out new information.

4. **Challenge yourself.** Mental stimulation is essential for keeping your mind sharp. By challenging yourself with new tasks and problems, you can keep your mind active and engaged.

5. **Take care of your body**. Your physical health has a direct impact on your mental health, so be sure to take care of yourself physically as well as mentally.

6. **Get enough sleep**: Most people need around eight hours of sleep per night.

7. **Eat healthily:** Eating a balanced diet helps your body and brain function at their best.

8. **Exercise:** Exercise releases endorphins, which have mood-boosting effects.

9. **Take breaks**: When you're feeling overwhelmed, take a few minutes to yourself to relax and de-stress.

The benefits of intellectual well being

It is widely accepted that there are numerous benefits to be gained from maintaining good intellectual health. These benefits range from improved cognitive functioning and memory to decreased risk of developing dementia later in life.

Furthermore, those who engage in activities that stimulate their minds on a regular basis are also more likely to experience a better quality of life overall.

Some of the specific benefits that have been linked to intellectual well-being include:

1. Improved cognitive functioning

As we age, it is natural for our cognitive abilities to decline. However, research has shown that those who engage in activities that stimulate their minds on a regular basis are able to slow down this process.

2. Improved memory

Like cognitive functioning, our memory also naturally deteriorates as we age. However, those who keep their minds active and challenged are able to delay the onset of memory problems.

3. Decreased risk of developing dementia

Dementia is a debilitating condition that can have a significant impact on an individual's quality of life. Research has shown that those who engage in intellectually stimulating activities are at a reduced risk of developing dementia later in life.

4. Increased sense of self-worth and purpose

Those who maintain good intellectual health often have a stronger sense of self-worth and purpose in life. This is because they feel like they are constantly learning and growing, which can lead to increased confidence and satisfaction with life in general.

5. **Improved mental and emotional health**

Intellectual well-being has also been linked to improved mental and emotional health. This is likely due to the fact that those who engage in intellectually stimulating activities often have increased levels of serotonin, which is a neurotransmitter that plays a role in mood regulation.

6. **Increased life satisfaction and happiness**

Finally, research has shown that those who maintain good intellectual health often report higher levels of life satisfaction and happiness. This is likely due to the fact that they feel like they are constantly learning and growing, which can lead to increased satisfaction with life in general.

In conclusion, there are many benefits to be gained from maintaining good intellectual health. These benefits include improved cognitive functioning, decreased risk of developing dementia, and increased life satisfaction.

Conclusion

Intellectual well-being is a state of being in which a person's intellectual needs are met and they are able to think critically and creatively. A person with intellectual well-being is curious and open-minded and has a growth mindset. They are also able to manage their emotions, set and achieve goals, and deal with stress in healthy ways.

There are many different ways to develop intellectual well-being. Certain things, however, are more significant than others. Reading, writing, being curious, challenging yourself, and taking care of your body are all great ways to improve your intellectual well-being.

There is no one-size-fits-all answer to the question of how to develop intellectual well-being. However, there are some key things that you can do to help yourself in this regard.

Firstly, make sure that you engage in activities that challenge your mind on a regular basis. This could involve anything from reading complex books to working on difficult puzzles.

Secondly, try to surround yourself with people who are stimulating and intellectually curious, as this will encourage you to think more deeply about the world around you.

Finally, don't be afraid to ask questions and seek out new information; the more you know, the easier it will be to develop a well-rounded understanding of the world and everything in it.

Intellectual wellness is important for both an individual and society. That said, there are many ways to improve it. One of the most important things is to regularly read, write, be curious, challenge yourself, and take care of your body.

Spending time with people who challenge your thinking and help you grow intellectually is also important. By following these tips and optimizing your actions, you can cultivate a rich inner life that will lead to a fulfilling existence.

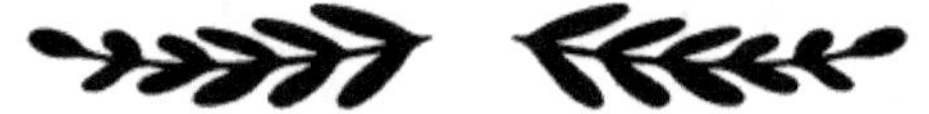

CHAPTER FOUR

IMPROVE MENTAL HEALTH

LIFESTYLE CHANGES

*"**M**ENTAL HEALTH...IS NOT A destination, but a process. It's about how you drive, not where you're going." —* Noam Shpancer, PhD

As the world becomes increasingly fast-paced and stressful, it's no wonder that mental health is becoming a bigger issue. The World Health Organization defines mental health as "a condition of well-being in which each individual fulfils his or her own potential, can cope with the usual demands of life, can work successfully and fruitfully, and is able to contribute to her or his community."

But what does this signify for those who are suffering from mental illness? What can people do to improve their well-being? In this blog post, we will look at several ways to improve your mental health.. From lifestyle changes to therapy and medication, there are many options available for those who want to improve their mental health.

One of the most important things you can do for your mental health is to adopt healthy lifestyle habits. Eating a nutritious diet, exercising regularly, getting enough sleep, and managing stress can all help improve mental health. Additionally, avoiding alcohol and drugs can also help reduce symptoms of mental illness.

Therapy

Another way to improve mental health is to seek out therapy. Talking to a therapist can help you work through difficult emotions, learn coping skills, and develop healthy thought patterns. Therapy can be an effective treatment for many mental health conditions, such as anxiety, depression, and post-traumatic stress disorder (PTSD).

Medication

For some people with mental illness, medication may be necessary in addition to therapy. Medication can help reduce symptoms of mental illness and allow people to better manage their condition. If you are considering medication for your mental health, it's important to speak with a doctor or psychiatrist to find out if it's right for you.

Self-care

Self-care is an important part of mental health. Taking care of yourself emotionally and mentally can help prevent or manage symptoms of mental illness. Some self-care activities include journaling, spending time in nature, practising meditation or mindfulness, and spending time with friends and family.

No matter what steps you take to improve your mental health, it's important to remember that help is available if you need it. If you are struggling to cope with your mental health, reach out to a doctor, therapist, or other mental health professional for help.

Identify Your Triggers

A trigger is anything that can bring on a bout of mental illness or make symptoms worse. Triggers can be external, like a stressful event, or internal, like negative thoughts.

Identifying your triggers is an important step in managing your mental health. Once you know what triggers your symptoms, you can develop a plan to avoid or cope with them.

There are many different ways to identify your triggers. Keeping a journal is one popular method. Every time you have a symptom or episode, write down what happened in the days leading up to it. Over time, you may start to see patterns emerge.

Another way to identify triggers is to talk to a therapist or counsellor. They can help you explore your past and present experiences to look for patterns and develop coping strategies.

Common triggers for mental illness include:

Stressful life events, such as a job loss or the death of a loved one

Trauma, such as physical or sexual abuse

Substance abuse

Relationship problems

Loneliness or social isolation

Certain medical conditions, such as thyroid problems or sleep disorders.

If you're not sure what's triggering your symptoms, talk to a mental health professional. They can help you explore your thoughts, feelings, and experiences to identify possible triggers.

Seek Out Supportive Relationships

When it comes to improving mental health, one of the best things you can do is seek out supportive relationships. These people will be there for you when times are tough, and

Get Moving

Exercise is a powerful tool for improving mental health. It can help reduce stress, improve sleep, and boost self-esteem. Exercise also causes the release of endorphins, which have mood-boosting properties.

To reap the benefits of exercise, you do not need to join a gym or begin training for a marathon. Just adding some activity to your day can make a big difference. Taking a brisk walk in the park, going for a bike ride, or even doing some yard work are all great ways to get moving.

Eat Right

What you eat has a big impact on your mental health. Eating a healthy diet can help improve mood, reduce anxiety and depression, and increase energy levels. On the other hand, eating an unhealthy diet can do the opposite.

To eat right, focus on consuming plenty of fruits, vegetables, whole grains, and lean protein. Also, limit sugary drinks and foods high in saturated fat. These simple changes can make a big difference in how you feel mentally and physically and will help you celebrate your successes. They're also the people who will challenge you to be your best self.

Supportive relationships can come from family, friends, co-workers, or even strangers. It's important to find people who make you feel good about yourself and whom you can rely on. When you have these types of relationships in your life, you'll feel more connected, supported, and loved—all of which are critical for maintaining good mental health.

Develop Healthy Coping Mechanisms

It is important to develop healthy coping mechanisms to improve mental health. Some unhealthy coping mechanisms include using drugs or alcohol to cope with stress, avoidance, numbing out with television or social media, and self-harm.

Healthy coping mechanisms are important because they help reduce stress and provide a sense of control. Some healthy coping mechanisms include exercise, journaling, talking to friends or family, meditation, and spending time in nature. Try out different coping mechanisms to see what works best for you.

Get Help When Needed

If you are struggling with your mental health, it is important to get help. Talk to your doctor or mental health professional about what you are going through. They can provide you with resources and support. There are also many hotlines and helplines available if you need someone to talk to. Don't be afraid to reach out for help when you need it.

Take care of yourself and don't be afraid to ask for help when needed.

Seek Professional Help When Needed

It's important to seek professional help when needed in order to improve mental health. There are many resources available to help individuals cope with mental health issues. Mental health professionals can provide guidance and support to help people manage their mental health.

Take care of your physical health

Your physical health is just as important as your mental health. Taking care of your body can help improve your mental health and vice versa.

Here are some tips to help you take care of your physical health:

- Get plenty of sleep: Most people need around eight hours of sleep per night. Getting enough sleep can help improve your mood, energy levels, and concentration.

- Eat a healthy diet: Eating healthy foods can help improve your mood and energy levels. Make sure to include plenty of fruits, vegetables, and whole grains in your diet.

- Exercise regularly: Exercise can help reduce stress, improve sleep, and boost your mood and energy levels. A moderate amount of exercise is the key to maintaining good physical health.

- See your doctor regularly: Seeing your doctor for regular check-ups can help catch any potential health problems early on.

Conclusion

If you're looking for ways to improve your mental health, there are a number of things you can do. From getting regular exercise and making sure you're getting enough sleep, to eating a healthy diet and spending time with supportive people, you can take many small steps that will make a big difference. Remember, it's important to be kind to yourself – give yourself time and space to heal, and don't hesitate to ask for help when you need it.

CHAPTER FIVE

HOW TO PRACTICE MINDFULNESS

HOW TO BE MINDFUL

"*MINDFULNESS IS A WAY of befriending ourselves and our experience*" - Jon Kabat-Zinn

When you think of mindfulness, what comes to mind? For many people, it conjures up images of sitting cross-legged on a cushion, eyes closed, with a peaceful look on their faces. While this is one way to practice mindfulness, it's not the only way.

Mindfulness is simply the act of paying attention to the present moment, without judgment. That means being aware of your thoughts, feelings, and sensations without getting caught up in them. It sounds easy enough, but in our fast-paced, constantly-connected world, it's harder than it seems.

The good news is that mindfulness is a skill that can be learned by anyone. And there are countless benefits to practicing mindfulness, including reducing stress and anxiety, improving sleep, and increasing focus and productivity.

So how do you get started? Below are some tips on how to practice mindfulness in your everyday life:

1. Set aside some time each day for mindfulness. Even just 5-10 minutes can make a difference.

2. Find a comfortable place to sit or lie down. You can close your eyes if you want, but it's not necessary.

3. Start focusing on your breath. Notice the sensation of the air moving in and out of your lungs. If your mind starts to wander (which it will!), simply bring your attention back to your breath.

4. Don't worry about doing it perfectly – there is no "right" way to meditate. Just let go of any expectations and be patient with yourself.

5. Remember that mindfulness is a practice, and like any skill, it takes time and effort to master. But with a little bit of practice, you'll be on your way to a more mindful life!

Mindfulness is the practice of paying attention to the present moment, without judgment. It can be helpful in managing stress, anxiety, and depression.

There are many ways to be mindful. One way is to focus on your breath. Pay attention to the sensation of the breath as it enters and leaves your body. Notice how your body feels as you breathe. Another way to be mindful is to focus on your senses. Notice what you see, hear, smell, taste, and feel.

Pay attention to the sensations in your body. You can also bring mindfulness into your daily activities by paying attention to what you are doing while you are doing it. For example, when you are eating, pay attention to the taste and texture of the food, and notice how your body feels as you eat.

You can also practice mindfulness through meditation. There are many different types of meditation, but one simple way to meditate is to sit quietly and focus on your breath. You may also want to try a guided meditation or a mindfulness app.

The important thing is to find a way that works for you and that you can stick with. Mindfulness takes practice, so be patient with yourself and keep at it!

The benefits of mindfulness

Mindfulness has many benefits, including reducing stress, improving focus and concentration, and promoting a sense of well-being.

In the workplace, mindfulness can help employees be more productive, creative, and efficient. It can also reduce work-related stress and burnout.

A growing body of research supports the benefits of mindfulness in the workplace. A recent study found that mindfulness training can help employees be more engaged and productive at work.

Another study found that mindfulness can help reduce job burnout and promote well-being in the workplace.

Mindfulness can also help leaders be more effective. A study of senior executives found that those who practiced mindfulness had lower levels of stress and better work-life balance.

How to practice mindfulness at work

There are many ways to incorporate mindfulness into your workday. Here are a few tips:

1. Make time for mindfulness. Schedule some time each day for mindfulness practice, even if it's just a few minutes.

2. Find a comfortable place to sit or stand. Close your eyes and focus on your breath.

3. Pay attention to your thoughts and emotions, but don't judge them. Let them come and go without clinging to them.

4. Return to your breath whenever your mind wanders.

5. Practice regularly, and you'll see the benefits in your work and in your life.

Mindfulness can be practised anywhere, at any time. It doesn't require special equipment or a lot of time. And it's something you can do on your own or with a group.

If you're new to mindfulness, there are many resources available to help you get started, including books, apps, and online courses.

Mindfulness ultimately is a state of being present in the moment, without judgment. It's an awareness that comes from paying attention to your thoughts, emotions, and sensations in the present moment.

When you're mindful, you're not trying to change anything or achieve anything. You're simply observing and accepting what is. This can be a difficult concept to grasp, but with practice, it can be very liberating.

Mindfulness can be practised in many ways, but a common thread is the focus on your breath. You can sit or lie down in a comfortable position and close your eyes. Then, simply pay attention to your breath as it goes in and out.

Your mind will inevitably wander, but that's okay. When you notice that your thoughts have drifted, simply bring your attention back to your breath.

With regular practice, you'll find that you're able to be more present and less reactive to the stresses of daily life. You may also find that you sleep better, have more energy, and feel calmer and more balanced.

The different types of mindfulness

Mindfulness can be practised in many different ways, each with its own benefits. Here are four popular types of mindfulness:

1. Formal mindfulness meditation involves sitting quietly and focusing on your breath, thoughts, or body sensations. This type of mindfulness can help you learn to control and focus your thoughts, as well as reduce stress and anxiety.

2. Body scan mindfulness is a type of mindfulness that involves paying attention to different parts of your body, from your toes to your head. This can help you become more aware of your body and any tension or pain you may be holding in specific areas.

3. Walking mindfulness involves paying attention to your surroundings and the sensation of walking while you walk. This can help you appreciate the world around you and get some exercise at the same time!

4. Eating mindfulness is all about being present and aware while you eat. This means savouring each bite, noticing the flavours and textures, and not letting yourself get distracted by other things going on around you. Eating mindfully can help you enjoy your food more and be more mindful of what you're putting into your body.

Mindfulness can be practiced in many different ways, each with its own benefits. Formal mindfulness meditation, body scan mindfulness, walking mindfulness, and eating mindfulness are all popular types of mindfulness that can help you reduce stress, anxiety, and pain, as well as improve your focus and concentration.

How to get started with mindfulness

If you're interested in mindfulness but aren't quite sure how to get started, this section is for you. Below, we'll provide some tips on how you can begin practising mindfulness in your everyday life.

1. Pay attention to your breath: One of the simplest and most effective ways to start practising mindfulness is to focus on your breath. When you find your mind wandering, simply bring your attention back to your breath and the sensation of air moving in and out of your body.

2. Observe your thoughts: Another key component of mindfulness is observing your thoughts without judgment. This means allowing yourself to notice whatever thoughts or emotions arise without getting caught up in them. Just let them come and go without attaching any importance to them.

3. Be present in the moment: Mindfulness also involves being present in the moment and not letting your mind wander off into the past or future. This means savouring each moment and really paying attention to what's happening around you, whether it's the taste of food, the sound of birds chirping, or the feel of a cool breeze on your skin.

4. Accept things as they are: Mindfulness also involves accepting things as they are, rather than trying to change them or resist them. This doesn't mean that you have to like everything that's happening, but it does mean accepting it non-judgmentally and letting go of any attached aversion or attachment.

5. Let go of perfectionism: Mindfulness can also help you let go of perfectionism by accepting that things are always changing and that there is no such thing as perfect. imperfections are part of life and trying to be perfect only leads to frustration, anxiety, and stress.

6. Be kind to yourself: One of the most important aspects of mindfulness is self-compassion. This means being kind and understanding towards yourself, even when you make mistakes or have negative thoughts or emotions. Remember that everyone makes mistakes and that you're just human.

7. Practice regularly: Like anything else, mindfulness takes practice. The more you practice, the easier it will become and the more benefits you'll experience. So don't be discouraged if it feels difficult at first. Just keep at it and eventually it will become second nature.

Mindfulness is a simple but powerful practice that anyone can benefit from. By paying attention to your breath, thoughts, and emotions, and accepting things as they are, you can learn to live in the present moment and find more peace and happiness in your life.

Conclusion

Mindfulness meditation is a form of mindfulness that can be practised anywhere, at any time.

All you need is a comfortable place to sit or recline, and the willingness to focus your attention on your breath and the present moment.

With regular practice, mindfulness meditation can help you learn how to better control your thoughts and emotions, and improve your overall well-being.

If you're interested in mindfulness but aren't quite sure how to get started, there are many resources available to help you, including books, apps, and online courses. The important thing is to find a way that works for you and that you can stick with. Mindfulness takes practice, so be patient with yourself and keep at it!

Mindfulness is a state of being present in the moment, without judgment. It's an awareness that comes from paying attention to your thoughts, emotions, and sensations in the present moment.

When you're mindful, you're not trying to change anything or achieve anything. You're simply observing and accepting what is. This can be a difficult concept to grasp, but with practice, it can be very liberating.

There are many benefits to practising mindfulness, including reducing stress, improving focus and concentration, promoting a sense of well-being, and more.

If you're interested in incorporating mindfulness into your life, there are many ways to do so, including formal mindfulness meditation, body scan mindfulness, walking mindfulness, and eating mindfulness.

The important thing is to find a way that works for you and that you can stick with. Mindfulness takes practice, so be patient with yourself and keep at it!

Mindfulness can be a difficult concept to grasp, but with practice, it can be very liberating.

There are many benefits to practising mindfulness, including reducing stress, improving focus and concentration, promoting a sense of well-being, and more.

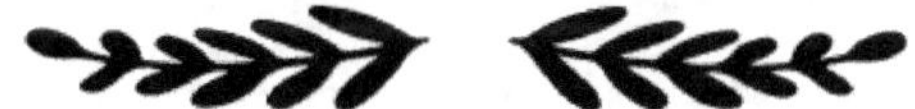

CHAPTER SIX

IMPROVE FOCUS AND CONCENTRATION

UNDERSTAND YOUR BRAIN

"Whenever you want to achieve something, keep your eyes open, concentrate and make sure you know exactly what it is you want. No one can hit their target with their eyes closed."- Paulo Coelho

You're trying to focus on your work, but your mind keeps wandering. You want to be productive, but you can't seem to get anything done. Sound familiar? It's normal for our attention spans to wander from time to time. But if you find that you can't focus on anything for more than a few minutes at a time, it might be time to take some action.

There are a number of things you can do to improve your focus and concentration. In this blog post, we'll explore some of the most effective methods and give you some tips on how to get started.

If you find that your attention span is wandering more often than not, it might be time to take some action to improve your focus and concentration. In this blog post, we'll explore some of the most effective methods for doing so, and give you some tips on how to get started.

Some of the most effective methods for improving focus and concentration include things like exercise, meditation, and getting enough sleep.

Exercise is a great way to improve focus and concentration. Not only does it help to get your blood flowing and your heart rate up, but it also can help to clear your mind and give you some time to think about something other than what's stressing you out.

Meditation is another excellent way to improve focus and concentration. It allows you to focus on your breath and clear your mind of any thoughts or worries that might be causing you stress.

Getting enough sleep is also critical for focus and concentration. When you're well-rested, you're able to think more clearly and have more energy to devote to whatever task you're trying to complete.

If you're finding it difficult to focus and concentrate, try implementing some of these methods into your daily routine. With a little bit of effort, you should see a significant improvement in your ability to focus and get things done.

Understand Your Brain

As we all know, the brain is a complex organ. It is responsible for our thoughts, emotions, and actions. So, it's no wonder that many of us struggle with focus and concentration at times.

But the good news is that there are things we can do to help improve our brain function. By understanding how our brains work, we can make small changes in our daily lives that can greatly impact our ability to focus and concentrate.

Here are some tips to help you understand your brain and improve your focus and concentration:

1. **Get enough sleep**: Sleep is crucial for brain health. When we don't get enough sleep, our brains have a harder time functioning properly. This can lead to problems with memory, Concentration difficulties were associated with decreased activity in the hippocampus and prefrontal cortex during waking hours., decision making, and emotional regulation.

So if you want to improve your focus and concentration, make sure you're getting enough shut-eye each night.

2. **Eat healthily**: What we eat affects our brains just as much as it affects the rest of our bodies. nutritious foods help the brain to function at its best while junk food can lead to problems with attention and focus. To keep your mind sharp, be sure to include plenty of healthy fats, proteins, vegetables, and whole grains in your diet.

3. **Exercise**: Exercise isn't just good for your body; it's also good for your brain.

4. **Take breaks**: When we focus on a task for too long, our brains become overwhelmed and we start to lose concentration. To avoid this, take breaks every 20 minutes or so to give your mind a chance to rest. During your break, you can do something calming like reading or taking a walk.

5. **Minimize distractions**: Our brains are easily distracted by things like noise, emails, and social media notifications. If you want to improve your focus, it's important to minimize distractions as much as possible. Turn off your phone, close your email browser, and find a quiet place to work.

6. **Practice mindfulness**: Mindfulness is the practice of being present in the moment and focusing on your breath. Research has shown that mindfulness can help improve attention and concentration .

7. **Get organized**: A cluttered environment can lead to a cluttered mind. So if you want to improve your focus, it's important to keep your workspace clean and organized. Make sure everything has its own place so you're not wasting time looking for things.

8. **Set goals**: When we have specific goals in mind, we're more likely to stay focused on the task at hand. So before starting a project, take a few minutes to think about what you want to achieve. This will help you stay on track and avoid getting side-tracked.

9. **Take your time**: Rushing through tasks can lead to mistakes and decreased concentration. So if you want to do your best work, it's important to take your time and focus on quality over quantity.

10. **Be patient**: Learning new things takes time and effort. Don't get discouraged if you don't understand something right away. Instead, be patient and give yourself time to learn. With practice, you'll eventually get the hang of it.

Stimulate Your Mind

There are a number of things you can do to stimulate your mind and improve your focus and concentration. Some simple tips include:

- Taking regular breaks from work or study to allow your mind to rest

- Getting plenty of sleep each night to ensure your brain is well-rested

- Eating a healthy diet to provide your body and brain with the nutrients it needs

- Exercising regularly to improve blood flow and oxygenation to the brain

- Practicing meditation or mindfulness techniques to help calm and focus the mind

By following these simple tips, you can help improve your focus and concentration levels, making it easier to get through even the most challenging tasks.

Get Moving

If you find yourself having trouble concentrating or focusing on a task, it may be time to get up and move your body. Research has shown that even a small amount of physical activity can help to improve focus and concentration.

So, if you're feeling sluggish or find yourself struggling to focus, take a break and get moving. Go for a walk, do some stretches, or jump up and down for a minute or two. You'll be surprised at how much better you feel and how much easier it is to concentrate after getting your body moving.

Reduce Distractions

Distractions are a major contributor to poor concentration and focus. If you're trying to get work done but find yourself constantly getting side-tracked by your phone, social media, or other distractions, it may be time to start working in a more distraction-free environment.

If possible, try working in a quiet room where you won't be interrupted by others or tempted to check your phone every five minutes. If you can't find a quiet place to work, try using noise-cancelling headphones or earplugs to help reduce distractions and improve your focus.

You should also try to limit the number of tasks you're working on at one time. Trying to juggle too many things at once will only make it harder to focus on any one task. So, if you have multiple projects that need your attention, take some time to prioritize and focus on one thing at a time.

Get Plenty of Sleep

It may seem obvious, but getting enough sleep is essential for concentration and focus. When you don't get enough sleep, it can be difficult to focus on anything. You may find yourself feeling irritable or anxious, and your memory and cognitive function may suffer.

If you're having trouble sleeping, there are a few things you can do to help improve your sleep quality. First, avoid caffeine and alcohol before bed. Both of these substances can interfere with sleep and make it harder to fall asleep or stay asleep throughout the night.

You should also create a relaxing bedtime routine that will help signal to your body that it's time to wind down for the night. This could include taking a warm bath, reading a book, or stretching before bed.

Finally, make sure your bedroom is dark, quiet, and cool—all of which can help promote better sleep.

Practice Meditation or Mindfulness

Meditation and mindfulness are both effective tools for improving concentration and focus. Meditation helps to train your attention span and improve your ability to focus on one thing at a time. Mindfulness, on the other hand, helps you to be more aware of the present moment and less likely to get distracted by thoughts or emotions that may pull your attention away from what you're trying to focus on.

Both meditation and mindfulness can be practised anywhere and don't require any special equipment.

There are many different meditation and mindfulness apps available that can help you get started. A headspace is a popular option that offers both guided and unguided meditation, while Calm is another good choice for beginners.

Give These Tips a Try

If you're having trouble concentrating or focusing, give these tips a try. By making some simple changes to your routine, you can improve your focus and concentration and get more done.

Improve Your Diet

If you want to improve your focus and concentration, one of the best things you can do is to improve your diet. Eating healthy foods that are rich in nutrients will help your brain to function at its best.

Some of the best foods for improving focus and concentration include:

1. **Omega-3 fatty acids**: These are found in oily fish like salmon, mackerel, and sardines, as well as in flaxseeds, chia seeds, and walnuts. Omega-3 fats are important for brain health and have been shown to improve cognitive function.

2. **Blueberries**: These delicious berries are packed with antioxidants and have been shown to boost cognitive function and memory.

3. **Green leafy vegetables**: Spinach, kale, and other green leafy vegetables are rich in vitamins and minerals that are essential for brain health. They also contain lutein, a compound that has been linked to improved cognition.

4. **Nuts and seeds**: Almonds, pistachios, sunflower seeds, and other nuts and seeds are excellent sources of protein, healthy fats, vitamins, minerals, and antioxidants. All of these nutrients are important for brain health and can help to improve focus and concentration.

5. **Dark chocolate**: Chocolate contains caffeine as well as flavonoids, which are compounds that have been shown to boost cognitive function. Choose dark chocolate with a high cocoa content for the most benefits.

Get Plenty of Sleep

Most people need around eight hours of sleep per night. However, some people may need more or less sleep depending on their age, lifestyle, and health. Sleep is essential for brain health and cognitive function. When you don't get enough sleep, it can affect your ability to focus and concentrate.

Aim to get 7-8 hours of sleep every night. If you have trouble sleeping, there are a few things you can do to improve your sleep quality:

1. Establish a regular sleep schedule by going to bed and waking up at the same time every day.

2. Avoid caffeine in the afternoon and evening.

3. Avoid working or using electronic devices in bed.

. Create a relaxing bedtime routine including winding down for 30 minutes before sleep.

5. Keep your bedroom dark, quiet, and cool.

Manage Stress

1. **Understand what stresses you out:** Everyone experiences stress differently, so it's important to understand what causes you to feel stressed. Identify your personal stressors and find healthy ways to cope with them.

2. **Make time for relaxation**: It's important to schedule time for relaxation and fun activities that help you de-stress. Whether it's reading, going for a walk, or taking a yoga class, make sure to give yourself some time to unwind.

3. **Stay healthy**: Eating healthy foods, exercising, and getting enough sleep are all crucial for managing stress levels. When your body is healthy, you're better able to handle stressors that come your way.

4. **Practice deep breathing**: Deep breathing is a simple yet effective way to instantly reduce stress levels. Whenever you're feeling overwhelmed, take a few minutes to focus on your breath and breathe deeply from your stomach.

5. **Connect with others**: Spending time with loved ones or close friends can help reduce stress levels. Talking about your worries with someone who cares can be a huge relief and help you better manage your stressors.

6. **Seek professional help**: If you're struggling to cope with stress on your own, don't hesitate to seek professional help. A therapist can assist you in identifying and managing your stressors in a healthy way.

Practice Relaxation Techniques

There are a number of different relaxation techniques that can help improve focus and concentration. Some popular techniques include:

1. **Breathing exercises** - Focus on taking deep, slow breaths and count to four as you inhale and exhale. This can help to clear your mind and relax your body.

2. **Muscle relaxation** - Start by tensing up your muscles as much as possible and then slowly releasing the tension. Focus on relaxing each muscle group one at a time.

3. **Imagery or visualization** - Picture yourself in a calm, relaxing setting such as lying on a beach or floating in a pool. Visualize all the stress leaving your body as you take deep breaths in and out.

4. **Meditation** - Sit quietly and focus on your breath going in and out of your body. Try to clear your mind of all thoughts and just focus on the present moment.

5. **Yoga or Tai Chi** - These mind-body practices can help to improve focus and concentration while also reducing stress levels.

Get regular exercise

Exercise is a great way to reduce stress and improve your overall health. It can also help you sleep better.

Eat a healthy diet

Eating a healthy diet can help your body function properly and reduce your risk for health problems.

There are a few things you can do to make sure you're getting enough sleep:

-Stick to a regular sleep schedule as much as possible.

-Create a calming bedtime routine to help you relax before sleep.

-Make sure your bedroom is dark, quiet, and cool.

-Limit screen time before bed.

-Avoid caffeine and alcohol before bed.

Take Breaks and Reward Yourself

It can be difficult to maintain focus and concentration for extended periods of time, but it is important to take breaks and reward yourself in order to stay on track. Here are a few tips:

1. Get up and move around every 20 minutes or so. This will help keep your energy levels up and prevent you from getting too comfortable in one position.

2. Set aside some time each day for a relaxing activity that you enjoy, such as reading, listening to music, or taking a bath.

3. Make sure to eat healthy foods and drink plenty of water throughout the day to keep your body and mind fuelled.

4. Take breaks regularly to stretch your legs, take deep breaths, or meditate for a few minutes.

5. Give yourself small rewards for completing tasks or staying focused for extended periods of time. This could be something as simple as taking a break to walk outside or enjoying a piece of chocolate.

Keeping a positive attitude and being patient with yourself are also important when trying to improve your focus. Remember that it takes time and practice to develop new habits, so be sure to be gentle with yourself during the learning process.

Conclusion

There are a number of ways to improve focus and concentration, and it really depends on what works best for you. Some people find that listening to music or white noise helps them to focus, while others prefer complete silence. Some people like to work in short bursts with frequent breaks, while others can maintain their focus for hours at a time.

Experiment with different techniques and find what works best for you. And remember, even if you can't always maintain perfect focus, don't be too hard on yourself - we all have our off days!

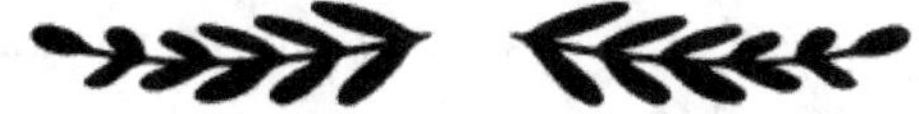

CHAPTER SEVEN

BEST RELAXATION TECHNIQUES

RELAXATION TECHNIQUES OVERVIEW

*"**J**UST TRUE TO FORM with life sometimes - what you're trying to do doesn't necessarily work out, but what ends up happening can be a lot better. I just relax and say whatever is going to happen – happens".*

Relaxation techniques are a form of self-care that can help reduce stress, and anxiety, and promote overall well-being. There are many different relaxation techniques that can be used, and finding the right one for you may take some trial and error. We will explore some of the most popular relaxation techniques and offer tips on how to get started. From deep breathing exercises to yoga and meditation, there are many ways to promote Relaxation. So, find what works best for you and start reaping the benefits today!

If you're like most people, chances are you don't make relaxation a priority. But what if I told you that relaxation is one of the keys to a happy and healthy life?

It's important to find what works best for you when it comes to relaxation techniques. We will explore some of the most popular relaxation techniques and offer tips on how to get started.

There are many relaxation techniques that can be useful in managing stress and anxiety. Some common relaxation techniques include:

-Deep breathing: Deep breathing is a simple but effective relaxation technique that can be done anywhere. Simply take a deep breath in through your nose, filling your lungs as much as possible. Then slowly exhale through your mouth. Repeat this several times.

-Progressive muscle relaxation: This technique involves tensing and relaxing different muscle groups in the body, one at a time. Start by tensing the muscles in your toes for a few seconds, then relax them. Work your way up the body, tensing and relaxing muscles group by group until you reach your head and neck.

-**Visualization:** Visualization involves picturing a peaceful or calming scene in your mind. It can help to focus on specific details, such as the colours of the scene, the sounds you hear, or the sensations you feel.

-**Yoga: Yoga** combines physical activity with breathing exercises and relaxation techniques. There are many different types of yoga, so it's important to find one that's right for you.

-**Tai chi**: Tai chi is a Chinese martial art that involves slow, graceful movements and deep breathing. Like yoga, tai chi can help to reduce stress and improve overall health.

-**Meditation:** Meditation involves focusing your attention on a specific object, thought, or activity. It can help to clear your mind and improve your focus.

Relaxation techniques can be used on their own or as part of a larger stress management plan.

Breathing exercises

Breathing exercises are a great way to relax and de-stress. There are many different breathing exercises you can do, but some of the most effective ones are diaphragmatic breathing, progressive muscle relaxation, and controlled breathing.

Diaphragmatic breathing is a great way to reduce stress and promote relaxation. To do this exercise, sit in a comfortable position with your back straight and your shoulders relaxed. Place one hand on your stomach just below your belly button. Slowly inhale through your nose, allowing your stomach to expand as you fill your lungs with air. As you exhale through your mouth, purse your lips and push all the air out of your lungs until your stomach contracts. Repeat this process for 10-15 minutes.

Controlled breathing is another simple but effective relaxation technique that can be done anywhere at any time. To do this exercise, simply breathe in through your nose for a count of four.

Breathe out through your mouth for a count of four. Repeat this process for 10-15 minutes.

Guided imagery

Guided imagery is a relaxation technique that involves using your imagination to create peaceful images in your mind. This exercise can be done anywhere at any time and is a great way to reduce stress and promote relaxation. To do this exercise, sit or lie down in a comfortable position and close your eyes.

Take a few deep breaths and focus on the image you want to create in your mind. It can be anything from a tranquil scene in nature to a calm, safe place. Once you have the image in your mind, focus on the details and try to make it as realistic as possible. Stay focused on the image for 5-10 minutes before opening your eyes and taking a few deep breaths.

Mindfulness meditation

Mindfulness meditation is a great way to focus on the present moment and let go of stress and anxiety. To do this exercise, find a comfortable place to sit or lie down. Close your eyes and take a few deep breaths. Focus on your breath and the sensations in your body. If your mind starts to wander, simply bring your attention back to your breath. Continue this process for 10-15 minutes.

Progressive muscle relaxation

Progressive muscle relaxation is another excellent way to reduce stress and promote relaxation. This exercise involves tensing and relaxing different muscle groups in the body. Start by tensing the muscles in your feet and ankles for 5-10 seconds before relaxing them completely. Then move up to your calves, thighs, hips, hands, arms, neck, and face, and tense each group of muscles for 5-10 seconds before relaxing them completely.

Once you've gone through all the muscle groups, take a few deep breaths and feel the tension leaving your body. Progressive muscle relaxation is a technique that can be used to relieve stress and tension. It involves the systematic tensing and relaxing of different muscle groups in the body.

This process can help to improve circulation, increase the range of motion, and reduce pain. It can also be used as a way to prepare for or recover from strenuous activity.

To do progressive muscle relaxation, start by sitting or lying in a comfortable position. Take a deep breath in and then exhale slowly. As you exhale, tense the muscles in your toes for 10 seconds. Then relax the muscles for 10 seconds as you breathe out.

Continue this pattern working your way up through each muscle group in your body: feet, calves, thighs, hips, abdomen, chest, arms, hands, neck, jaw, and face. Make sure to spend an equal amount of time tensing and relaxing each muscle group.

Visualization

There are a number of different visualization techniques that can be used for relaxation. One popular technique is to imagine a peaceful or calming scene, such as a beach or a forest. Other techniques include focusing on your breath and counting each inhale and exhale or picturing a relaxing colour or image.

Visualization can be used anywhere and at any time – you don't need any special equipment or environment. Simply close your eyes and focus on the image, scene or sensation you want to create in your mind. The more vivid and realistic you can make it, the more effective it will be.

Regular practice of visualization can help to reduce stress levels, improve sleep quality and increase overall feelings of well-being.

Aromatherapy

Aromatherapy is a form of alternative medicine that uses essential oils to promote relaxation and well-being. Aromatherapy can be used in a variety of ways, including inhalation and topical application.

The most popular essential oils used in aromatherapy include lavender, chamomile, and peppermint. These oils are believed to have properties that can help to relieve stress, anxiety, and tension. Aromatherapy is often used as a complementary treatment to other relaxation techniques, such as yoga or meditation.

Yoga

Yoga is a relaxation technique that can be used to ease the mind and body. Yoga poses, or asanas, are designed to stretch and tone the muscles, improve flexibility, and release tension. Breath work, or pranayama, is an important part of yoga and helps to control the breath and calm the mind. Meditation is another important element of yoga practice and can be used to focus the mind and promote inner peace.

Inhale as you return to the starting position. Exhale as you repeat the movement on the other side. Continue moving slowly and smoothly through the movements, focusing on your breath and body posture.

Tai chi

Tai chi is a Chinese martial art that involves slow, graceful movements and deep breathing. Tai chi can be done alone or in a group, and there is no need for any special equipment or clothing.

Regular practice of tai chi can help to reduce stress, improve balance and coordination, and increase flexibility and range of motion. Tai chi can also be used as a form of self-defence.

To do tai chi, start by standing with your feet shoulder-width apart and your arms at your sides. Slowly shift your weight to your left foot and raise your right hand in front of you, keeping your palm open. As you exhale, turn your palm to face downwards and sweep your hand down to your left side. Tai chi is a form of martial arts that originated in China.

It is based on the principle of using slow, controlled movements to achieve balance and harmony between the body and mind. Tai chi is often described as "meditation in motion" because it promotes re-laxation and stress relief.

There are many benefits of practising tai chi, including improved balance and coordination, reduced stress and anxiety, better sleep, and increased strength and flexibility. Tai chi can be done by people of all ages and fitness levels. It is a safe, low-impact form of exercise that can be done indoors or outdoors.

If you're looking for a way to relax and de-stress, tai chi may be a good option for you.

Meditation

Meditation is a popular relaxation technique that can be used to help reduce stress, anxiety, and tension. There are many different ways to meditate, so it's important to find a method that works best for you. One of the most common ways to meditate is to focus on your breath. Sit or lie down in a comfortable position and close your eyes.

Slowly inhale and exhale, paying attention to your breath as it enters and leaves your body. If your mind starts to wander, simply redirect your focus back to your breath. You can also try focusing on a mantra or word that you repeat to yourself during meditation.

Spending even a few minutes meditating can help to calm and focus the mind. With regular practice, meditation can help to reduce stress levels, improve sleep quality, and increase overall well-being.

Tips for choosing the right relaxation technique

There is no one-size-fits-all answer to this question, as the best relaxation technique for you may vary depending on your individual needs and preferences. However, there are a few key things to keep in mind when choosing a relaxation technique that will help you find the one that works best for you.

First, consider what you want to achieve through relaxation. Do you want to reduce stress, improve sleep, or boost your mood? Once you know what your goal is, you can narrow down your options and choose a technique that is best suited to help you achieve it.

Second, think about what type of environment you feel most relaxed in. Do you prefer being outdoors in nature, or indoors in a quiet room?

This will help guide you towards techniques that will be most effective for you.

Finally, consider your personal preferences and needs when choosing a relaxation technique. For example, if you have trouble sitting still, then a moving meditation like Tai Chi or Yoga might be a better option for you than something like mindfulness meditation. Trust your instincts and go with what feels right for you.

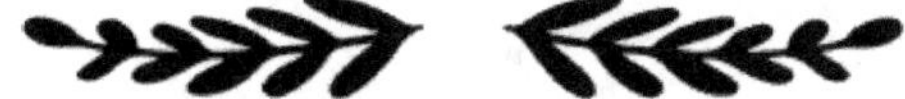

Take a Break

WE HAVE REACHED A mid point of the book. You may like to take a break and give a feedback on this book , in the form of a rating or a review on Amazon or Goodreads . This will help immensely in spreading the message in the reading community.

Besides, your suggestions are incredibly important to my creative process as an independent writer. It not only fuels my passion but also allows me to go deeply into the core of my creative attempts and find the very heart of my writing. I respectfully ask that you think about posting a review / rating for " **Mind Your Mind** " in order to gain your useful insights and opinions.

It is not necessary for your review to be in-depth or extensive; even a brief collection of ideas that expresses your true feelings will do. Whether your comments are compliments or constructive criticism, they all serve as important building bricks in my search for ongoing development as a writer and storyteller.

You might prefer to scan the QR Code below using your smart phone.

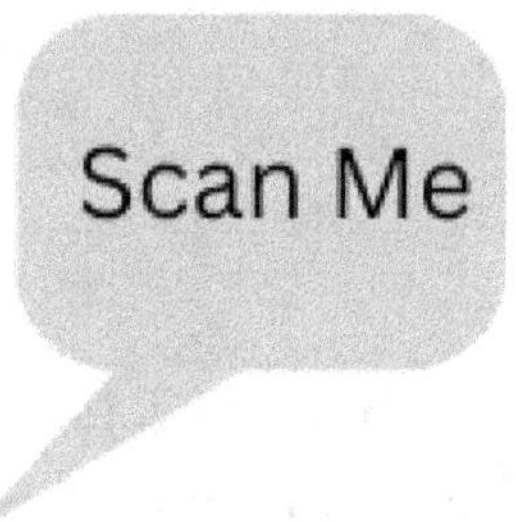

Scan QR Code with your smart phone a leave a review

CHAPTER EIGHT

BOOST YOUR MOOD

THE SCIENCE OF HAPPINESS

"**D**ON'T WORRY. JUST WHEN you think your life is over, a new storyline falls from the sky and lands right in your lap." — Rebekah Crane

We all have our down days. Maybe you're feeling stressed from work, or you're just not in the mood for anything. Whatever the reason, it's important to know how to boost your mood when you're feeling down. There are a few simple things you can do to turn that frown upside down. In this blog post, we'll explore some of the most effective ways to boost your mood and get you back on track. From exercise to diet and everything in between, read on for some tips on how to improve your mood today

The science of happiness is the study of what makes people happy and how to increase happiness levels. There are many different factors that can contribute to happiness, and scientists are constantly discovering new ones. Some of the most important factors include:

-having close relationships with family and friends

-feeling like you belong to a community or group

-having a sense of control over your life

-feeling competent and capable

-having a purpose or goal in life

There are also many things you can do to increase your happiness levels. Some simple tips include:

-expressing gratitude regularly

-performing acts of kindness

-taking time for leisure activities and relaxation

-investing time in relationships

-eating healthy foods

-exercising regularly

The Different Types of Happiness

It's no secret that happiness is the key to a good life. But what exactly is happiness? And what are the different types of happiness?

Happiness is a state of well-being characterized by positive emotions like joy, satisfaction, and contentment. There are different types of happiness, however, each with its own set of causes and effects.

The first type of happiness is hedonic happiness, which refers to the pleasure we feel from experiencing positive emotions and sensations. This type of happiness is often short-lived, as it depends on external factors that are beyond our control.

The second type of happiness is eudaimonia happiness, which refers to a more lasting sense of well-being that comes from achieving our personal goals and living a meaningful life. Eudemonic happiness requires effort and planning, but it leads to a more fulfilling and sustainable form of happiness.

No matter what type of happiness you're striving for, there are certain things you can do to boost your mood and increase your overall sense of well-being. Here are some tips:

Be positive

When it comes to mood boosters, being positive is key. No matter what life throws your way, try to stay upbeat and look on the bright side. Doing so will not only benefit your mood, but also your overall health. Here are a few ways to stay positive:

• Find things to be thankful for: Every day, take a few minutes to write down three things you're grateful for. This could be anything from your health to a great parking spot. Focusing on the positives in your life can help shift your perspective and make you feel happier.

• Be mindful of your thoughts: Pay attention to the negative thoughts running through your head and work on reframing them in a more positive light. Instead of dwelling on what went wrong, focus on what you can do to improve the situation.

• Smile more: It may sound clichéd, but smiling really is contagious. Not only will it make you feel better, but it could also brighten someone else's day.

• Help others: When you lend a helping hand, it can not only make someone else's day better but also boost your own mood. altruistic acts release endorphins in the brain, which have mood-lifting effects.

Find a creative outlet

When you're feeling down, it can be tough to find the motivation to do anything. However, one of the best ways to boost your mood is to find a creative outlet. Whether it's painting, writing, playing music, or another form of self-expression, getting your creative juices flowing can help you feel better.

Not only does being creative help you express yourself and explore your emotions, but it can also be a great way to distract yourself from whatever is stressing you out. When you're focused on creating something new, you're not as likely to dwell on negative thoughts. And even if you don't consider yourself "creative," there are still plenty of ways to get involved in some form of art. So next time you're feeling down, try one of these activities:

• Take a painting class

• Write in a journal

• Learn how to play an instrument

- Make a scrapbook

- Bake something new

Get active

Yes, endorphins are real. And, yes, they can help improve your mood. But how do you go about getting them?

The best way to get active and boost your mood is to find an activity that you enjoy and stick with it. It doesn't have to be a high-intensity workout; even moderate exercise can release endorphins. So take a walk, go for a bike ride, take a yoga class, or play your favorite sport. Just make sure to get moving for at least 30 minutes a day.

Connect with nature

There are many ways to boost your mood, but one of the most effective is to connect with nature. Spend time outside in the sun, fresh air, and natural scenery. Take a walk in the park or go for a hike in the woods. Let the sights, sounds, and smells of nature rejuvenate and refresh you.

When you're feeling stressed or down, take a break to appreciate the beauty of nature all around you. Go outside and take a deep breath. Notice the fresh air filling your lungs. Look up at the sky and appreciate the sunlight shining down on you. Listen to the birds singing or the leaves rustling in the wind. Smell the flowers or freshly cut grass. Touch a tree trunk or feel the softness of a petal.

Spending time in nature can help reduce stress, anxiety, and depression while improving moods and overall mental health. So next time you're feeling low, step outside and let nature work its magic!

Help others

When you help others, you forget your own troubles and feel good about yourself. It's a win-win situation! So the next time you're feeling down, do something nice for someone else.

You can help out a neighbor, volunteer at a local organization, or even just hold the door open for someone. Whatever you do, know that you're making a difference and boosting your mood in the process.

Final thoughts

If you're feeling down, there are plenty of things you can do to boost your mood. From getting active and spending time outside to helping others and being creative, there are many ways to feel better. So find what works for you and start feeling better today!

Make time for yourself

It's important to make time for yourself, even when you're feeling low. Taking some time out for yourself can help you boost your mood and give you some much-needed perspective.

One way to make time for yourself is to schedule it into your day. Make sure you set aside at least 30 minutes each day to do something that makes you happy. This could be reading, taking a walk, listening to music, or anything else that brings you joy.

If you find it difficult to stick to a schedule, try breaking up your day into smaller chunks of time. Dedicate 10 minutes here and there to doing something calming or fun. Once you get in the habit of taking some me-time, it will become easier and feel more natural.

Boosting your mood doesn't have to be complicated or time-consuming. By making a little bit of time for yourself each day, you can start feeling better in no time!

Conclusion

There are many ways to boost your mood, and it ultimately comes down to finding what works best for you. Experiment with different activities and strategies until you find a combination that works for you. And don't forget to give yourself some grace - sometimes feeling down is just a part of life. But by using these tips, you can hopefully increase the frequency of those good days.

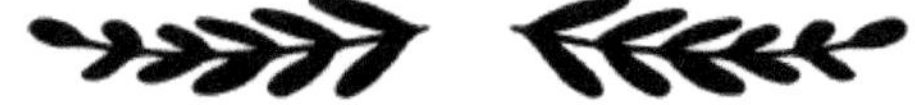

CHAPTER NINE

HAVE A POSITIVE MINDSET

"WE BECOME WHAT WE think about."

No matter what life throws your way, having a positive mindset can help you overcome any challenge. A positive mindset is a powerful tool that can help you achieve your goals and improve your overall well-being. If you're looking to improve your outlook on life, here are some tips on how to have a positive mindset.

Tip 1: Be mindful of your thoughts

Your thoughts play a big role in shaping your outlook on life. If you're constantly thinking negative thoughts, it's going to be difficult to have a positive outlook. Pay attention to the thoughts that run through your head and try to catch yourself when you're thinking something negative. Once you're aware of your negative thoughts, you can start to challenge them. Ask yourself if there's any evidence to support your negative thought. Most of the time, you'll find that there isn't.

Tip 2: Surround yourself with positive people

The people you spend time with can also influence your mindset. If you're around people who are always complaining or who see the glass as half empty, it's going to be tough to stay positive. Instead, try to surround yourself with people who have a positive outlook on life. These people will help remind you of the good in life and can provide support when you're feeling down.

Tip 3: Practice gratitude

Gratitude is another tool that can help you shift your mindset from negative to positive. When you take the time to appreciate the good in your life, it's easier to see the silver lining in difficult situations. Start each day by writing down three things you're grateful for. At the end of each week, reflect on five things that went well. This exercise will help train your brain to focus on the positive.

Tip 4: Take care of yourself

It's important to take care of yourself physically and emotionally if you want to maintain a positive mindset. Make sure you're getting enough sleep, eating healthy foods, and exercising regularly. It's also important to find ways to manage stress in a healthy way. Taking care of yourself will help you feel better both physically and mentally, which can positively impact your outlook on life.

Practising these tips can help you develop a more positive mindset. Having a positive outlook on life can improve your physical health, help you achieve your goals, and make you feel happier overall.

The power of positive thinking

You've heard it said that laughter is the best medicine. Well, it turns out that there may be some truth to that saying. According to a growing body of scientific evidence, positive thinking can improve our physical health as well as our mental and emotional well-being.

Positive thinking has been linked with lower rates of heart disease, less stress and anxiety, stronger immune systems, and increased life expectancy. In one study, people who had a positive outlook on life were found to live an average of 7.5 years longer than those who didn't have a positive outlook.

While we can't control everything that happens to us in life, we can control our attitude and how we react to the events that occur. So if you're looking for ways to improve your health and wellbeing, start by thinking more positively!

Here are some tips to get you started:

Focus on the positive. Make an effort to focus on the good things in your life, no matter how small they may seem. Each day, take a few minutes to write down three things that you're grateful for.

Make an effort to focus on the good things in your life, no matter how small they may seem. Each day, take a few minutes to write down three things that you're grateful for. Be mindful of your self-talk . The way we talk to ourselves can have a big impact on our outlook on life. If you find yourself constantly putting yourself down or dwelling on negative thoughts, make a conscious effort to change your self-talk. Instead of saying "I can't do this," try telling yourself "I can do this!"

. The way we talk to ourselves can have a big impact on our outlook on life. If you find yourself constantly putting yourself down or dwelling on negative thoughts, make a conscious effort to change your self-talk. Instead of saying "I can't do this," try telling yourself "I can do this!" Surround yourself with positive people. Spend time with people who make you feel good about yourself and who will support you in pursuing your goals.

Spend time with people who make you feel good about yourself and who will support you in pursuing your goals. Practice positive visualization. Visualize yourself achieving your goals and living the life you want. See yourself surrounded by the people and things that make you happy. The more vividly you can imagine it, the better!

Visualize yourself achieving your goals and living the life you want. See yourself surrounded by the people and things that make you happy. The more vividly you can imagine it, the better! Don't sweat the small stuff. Life is too short to worry about things that don't really matter in the grand scheme of things. So instead of getting worked up over every little thing that goes wrong, try to take a step back and perspective.

Making even a small effort to think more positively can have a big impact on your health and wellbeing. So why not give it a try?

Overcoming negative thoughts

Negative thinking is a common barrier to happiness and success. But it doesn't have to be this way! You can learn how to overcome negative thoughts and cultivate a more positive mindset.

Here are some tips for overcoming negative thoughts:

1. Acknowledge your negative thought. Don't try to ignore it or push it away. Accepting that you have a negative thought can be the first step to letting it go.

2. Examine your negative thought. Once you've acknowledged your negative thought, take a closer look at it. What is it really saying? Is there any truth to it? Or is it just an irrational fear?

3. Reframe your negative thought. If you find that there is some truth to your negative thought, try to reframe it in a more positive light. For

example, instead of "I'm not good enough," try "I'm doing my best and I will improve with time and practice."

4. Let go of your negative thought. Once you've examined and reframed your negative thought, it's time to let it go. Visualize yourself releasing the thought, or imagine putting it in a balloon and watching it float away into the sky.

5. Practice positive thinking. Make a conscious effort to focus on the positive things in your life. Each day, write down three things you're grateful for. Or, whenever you have a negative thought, counter it with a positive one.

Overcoming negative thoughts takes time and practice. But if you're patient and persistent, you can train your brain to think more positively!

Building a positive mindset

Building a positive mindset is not always easy. It takes time, effort and practice. However, it is worth it! A positive mindset can lead to a happier, healthier and more successful life.

Here are some tips for building a positive mindset:

1. Be mindful of your thoughts. What you think has a big impact on how you feel. Pay attention to your thoughts and try to make them more positive.

2. Practice gratitude. Be thankful for the good things in your life, no matter how small they may be. Gratitude will help you appreciate what you have and attract more good things into your life.

3. Take care of yourself. A healthy body and mind are essential for a positive outlook on life. Eat healthy foods, exercise regularly, get enough sleep and find ways to relax and de-stress.

4. Connect with others. Social support is crucial for our well-being. Spend time with family and friends, join groups or clubs with like-minded people, or volunteer in your community.

5. Do something nice for someone else. Helping others can make us feel good about ourselves and brighten someone else's day too!

6. Set realistic goals. Having something to strive for can give us a sense of purpose and motivation. Make sure your goals are achievable and realistic, so you can feel good about accomplishing them.

7. Find your "happy place". Everyone has a different activity or place that makes them feel happy and relaxed. It could be spending time in nature, listening to music, reading, playing with a pet, or anything else that brings you joy. Make time for your happy place every day!

8. Be patient. Rome wasn't built in a day and neither is a positive mindset. It takes time and effort to change the way you think, but it is possible. Be patient with yourself and keep working at it.

Building a positive mindset is not always easy, but it is worth it! These tips can help you get started on the path to a happier, healthier life.

The benefits of having a positive mindset

When it comes to having a positive outlook on life, the benefits are endless. A positive mindset can lead to increased happiness, better health, and improved relationships. Here are just a few of the ways that having a positive mindset can improve your life:

1. Increased happiness: People who have a positive outlook on life tend to be happier than those who don't. Why? Because they focus on the good in their lives instead of the bad. They also tend to have an optimistic view of the future, which leads to greater happiness overall.

2. Better health: Numerous studies have shown that people who have a positive attitude tend to be healthier than those with a negative outlook. This is likely due to the fact that positive people take better care of themselves and are more likely to adopt healthy lifestyle habits.

3. Improved relationships: Positive people are also more likely to have strong and healthy relationships than those with a negative mindset. This is because they exude confidence and warmth, which makes them more likeable and approachable. Additionally, positive people are less likely to dwell on past arguments or harbour resentment towards others.

4. Greater success: Finally, people with a positive mindset are more likely to achieve their goals than those with a negative outlook. This is because they believe in themselves and their ability to overcome obstacles. They also don't let setbacks or failures get them down, which allows them to keep moving forward towards their goals.

In conclusion, it's clear that there are many benefits to having a positive mindset. If you're looking to improve your life in any way, adopting a positive attitude is a great place to start.

Conclusion

Having a positive mindset is one of the most important things you can do for yourself. It's not always easy, but it's worth it. When you have a positive outlook on life, you're more likely to be successful, happy, and healthy. Here are a few tips to help you develop and maintain a positive mindset: 1. Be grateful for what you have. 2. Focus on the good in every situation. 3. Find humour in everyday situations. 4. Surround yourself with positive people. 5. Practice positive visualization. 6. Don't sweat the small stuff. 7. Take care of yourself physically and emotionally. 8. Be patient with yourself.

If you're looking to improve your life in any way, developing a positive mindset is a great place to start.

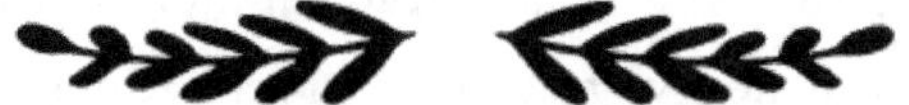

How to Identify Your Triggers

What is a Trigger?

"**A**LL PAIN TRIGGERS A reminder, deeper than thought, buzzing through blood and bone, that we are fragile and finite." —— K.J. Ramsey

We all have triggers. They are the things that set us off, make us react, or put us in a bad mood. And while we can't always control what happens to us, we can control how we react to it. Part of learning how to deal with our triggers is learning how to identify them.

Once we know what sets us off, we can begin to work on managing our reactions. In this blog post, we will explore how to identify your triggers and start working towards managing them. From keeping a journal to building self-awareness, read on for some tips on how you can better understand your triggers and take control of your reactions.

Do you often find yourself getting angry or upset and not knowing why? If you can't seem to pinpoint what sets you off, you're not alone. Many of us have triggers that we aren't aware of. Luckily, there are some things you can do to start identifying your triggers. Keep reading to learn more.

What is a trigger?

A trigger is a cue or event that sets off a memory or reaction in your brain. Triggers can be external, like a sight, sound, smell, taste, touch, place, or thing. They can also be internal, like a thought, feeling, or memory.

Some triggers are positive and cause you to feel happy or excited. Other triggers are negative and can cause you to feel angry, sad, anxious, or afraid.

Triggers can be intense and overwhelming. They can make you feel like you're back in the middle of the trauma or event that caused them. This can be extremely distressing and may even lead to flashbacks (intrusive memories), dissociation (feeling disconnected from your body), or panic attacks.

If you're struggling to manage your triggers, it's important to seek help from a mental health professional. They can provide you with tools and techniques to deal with triggers in a healthy way.

What are some examples of triggers?

There are endless possibilities when it comes to triggers. Here are a few examples:

• A sound that reminds you of a car accident you were in

• A smell that reminds you of the hospital where your loved one died

• A touch that reminds you of being sexually assaulted

• A place that reminds you of the war zone you were in

• A thing that reminds you of the house fire you survived

• A thought that reminds you of a failed test or relationship

Remember, everyone is different. What may be a trigger for one person may not be a trigger for another.

What are some coping skills for dealing with triggers?

There are many different coping skills that can help you deal with triggers in a healthy way. Some coping skills may work better for you than others. It's important to experiment and find what works best for you.

Here are a few examples of coping skills:

• Deep breathing

• Progressive muscle relaxation

• Visualization

• Mindfulness meditation

• Guided imagery

• Art therapy

• Music therapy

• Exercise

• Journaling

• Talking to a friend or therapist

Why are triggers important to identify?

Triggers are important to identify because they can help you to avoid stressful situations and to manage your stress more effectively. Triggers can be anything that makes you feel stressed, anxious, or angry. Some common triggers include:

-Certain people or places

-Certain situations or events

- Certain thoughts or memories

Identifying your triggers can help you to avoid them or to prepare for them in advance. This can make a big difference in your stress levels and in your ability to cope with difficult situations.

How to identify your triggers

One of the most difficult aspects of managing anxiety is understanding what triggers your anxious feelings. Everyone experiences anxiety differently, and what might trigger one person's anxiety may not trigger another person's anxiety. However, there are some general tips that can help you identify your own personal triggers.

Pay attention to your body: One of the first places to start when trying to identify your triggers is to pay attention to your body. Does your heart rate increase or do you start to feel shaky when you're in a certain situation? These physical cues can be clues that you're experiencing anxiety.

Think about your thoughts: Another clue that can help you identify your triggers is to think about the thoughts that run through your head when you're feeling anxious. Do you start to worry about things that might happen in the future? Do you replay past events in your mind? Identifying these negative thought patterns can help you understand what situations tend to trigger your anxiety.

Keep a journal: One of the best ways to identify your triggers is to keep a journal documenting when you feel anxious and what situations were going on around you at the time. This can help you see patterns in your behaviour and better understand what makes you feel anxious.

Talk to others: Talking to others who experience anxiety can also be helpful in identifying your own triggers. They may be able to share their experiences with you and offer insight into what might be triggering your anxiety.

If you're having trouble identifying your anxiety triggers, consider talking to a mental health professional. They can help you understand your anxiety and develop a plan to manage it.

Tips for managing anxiety triggers

Once you've identified your anxiety triggers, there are a number of things you can do to manage them. Here are a few tips:

Avoid your triggers: One of the best ways to manage your anxiety is to avoid the situations that trigger it. If you know that being in large crowds makes you feel anxious, try to avoid places like shopping malls or concerts.

Create a plan: If you can't avoid your anxiety triggers, it's important to have a plan for how you'll deal with them when they occur. This might involve deep breathing exercises, visualization, or positive self-talk. Having a plan in place can help you feel more prepared and less anxious when faced with a trigger.

Talk to someone: Talking to someone about your anxiety can also be helpful. This might be a friend, family member, therapist, or doctor.

Talking about your anxiety can help you better understand it and find ways to cope with it.

Know your limits: It's also important to know your limits when it comes to managing your anxiety. If you're feeling overwhelmed, don't hesitate to take a break or remove yourself from the situation. It's okay to take care of yourself and put your needs first.

Anxiety is a normal and common emotion that everyone experiences at times. However, for some people, anxiety can become so severe that it interferes with their daily lives. If you're struggling with anxiety, there are a number of things you can do to manage it. These include identifying your anxiety triggers, creating a plan for how to deal with them, and talking to someone about your anxiety.

Once you've identified your triggers, what do you do with that information?

Now that you know what sets off your triggers, it's time to do something about it. Here are a few ideas:

-Talk to someone who understands. This could be a therapist, counsellor, or trusted friend or family member. Just talking about what's going on can be helpful.

-Avoid the trigger if possible. If there's something you know sets off your anxiety, try to avoid it if at all possible.

-Challenge your thinking. If you find yourself getting anxious about something, ask yourself if there's evidence to support your fears. Often, we're more afraid of things than we need to be.

-Practice relaxation techniques. When you start to feel anxious, take some deep breaths and try to relax your body. There are also specific relaxation techniques like progressive muscle relaxation that can be helpful.

-Exercise. Physical activity can help reduce anxiety and make you feel better overall.

-Get enough sleep. Lack of sleep can make anxiety worse, so make sure you're getting enough rest.

-Talk to your doctor. If your anxiety is really severe, your doctor may be able to prescribe medication or refer you to a therapist.

If you're struggling with anxiety, don't hesitate to seek help. There are many resources available and you don't have to go through it alone.

Conclusion

Now that you know what a trigger is and how to identify your own, you can start to work on managing them. This may involve avoiding certain triggers altogether, or learning how to deal with them in a healthy way. If you're not sure where to start, talk to your doctor or a qualified mental health professional. They can help you develop a plan for dealing with your triggers and help you get on the road to recovery.

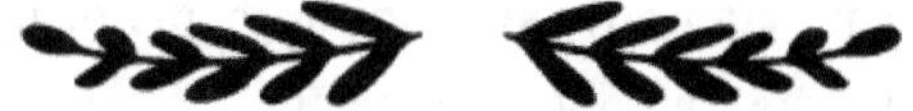

CHAPTER ELEVEN

WHAT IS MINDFUL MEDITATION?

"MEDITATION MEANS LETTING GO of our baggage, letting go of all the pre-rehearsed stories and inner-dialogue that we've grown so attached to." -, Headspace co-founder

Mindfulness meditation is a type of mindfulness practice that involves focusing your attention on your breath and being aware of your thoughts and sensations without judgment.

When you focus on your breath, you may notice that your mind wanders off. That's okay! Mindfulness is about noticing when your mind has wandered and gently bringing it back to the present moment.

There are many different ways to meditate, but mindfulness meditation is a good place to start if you're new to meditation. You can practice mindfulness meditation anywhere, at any time. All you need is a comfortable place to sit or lie down.

If you're interested in learning more about mindfulness meditation, there are many resources available online and in libraries. Once you've learned the basics, you may want to explore other types of meditation, such as loving-kindness meditation or mantra meditation.

The Benefits of Mindfulness Meditation

Mindfulness meditation has many benefits that can help improve your quality of life. Some of the benefits include:

1. Improving your focus and concentration

2. Reducing stress and anxiety

3. Helping to control impulses and motions

4. improving sleep quality

5. Boosting your immune system

6. Reducing pain

7. Improving your overall sense of well-being

How to Get Started with Mindfulness Meditation

If you're new to mindfulness meditation, it can be helpful to understand the basics of how to get started. The first step is to find a comfortable place to sit or recline in. You may want to close your eyes and focus on your breath.

Once you're settled, begin to pay attention to your breath. Notice the sensation of the air moving in and out of your lungs. Don't try to control your breath, simply let it flow naturally. If your mind begins to wander, gently bring your attention back to your breath.

You may also want to focus on other sensations in your body, such as the feel of your clothes against your skin or the sound of your heartbeat. Simply notice these things without judging them as good or bad.

Allow yourself to be aware of thoughts and emotions as they arise, but don't get caught up in them. Just let them come and go without judging them. If you find yourself getting lost in thought, simply return your attention to your breath or another sensation in your body.

Mindfulness meditation can be practiced for any length of time, but even a few minutes can be beneficial. Start with whatever amount of time feels comfortable for you and gradually increase it as you become more familiar with the practice.

There are many different ways to meditate, so experiment to find what works best for you. There are no right or wrong way to meditate, so just do what feels natural for you.

Tips for Practicing Mindfulness Meditation

Mindfulness meditation is a form of mindfulness that is widely practiced in the western world. There are many benefits to practicing mindfulness meditation, including reducing stress, improving mental and physical health, and increasing focus and concentration.

If you're interested in trying mindfulness meditation, here are a few tips to get started:

1. Find a comfortable place to sit or lie down. You don't need to be in a special position to meditate, just make sure you're comfortable so you can focus on your breath.

2. Close your eyes and focus on your breath. Once you're settled, take a few deep breaths and then focus on your breath as it gently moves in and out of your body.

3. Don't try to control your thoughts. One of the most difficult things about meditation is letting go of our constant stream of thoughts. Instead of trying to stop your thoughts altogether, simply observe them as they come and go without judgement.

4. Be patient with yourself. Meditation takes practice and there will be times when it's difficult to focus or keep your mind from wandering. Don't get discouraged – just keep coming back to your breath each time you notice your mind has wandered off.

5. Make it a daily practice. The more you meditate, the easier it will become. Try to make it a daily practice, even if it's just for a few minutes at a time.

Mindfulness meditation is a simple practice that can have a profound impact on your well-being. Give it a try and see how it goes!

Guided Mindfulness Meditation Practices

If you're new to mindfulness meditation, it can be helpful to have some guidance when you're getting started. There are many different ways to meditate, but all of them involve focusing your attention on the present moment and letting go of distractions.

One popular way to meditate is to focus on your breath. Start by finding a comfortable position and closing your eyes. Then, simply notice the sensation of your breath as you inhale and exhale. If your mind starts to wander, gently bring it back to your breath. You can also try counting each breath or focusing on a mantra or word that you repeat to yourself.

Another common practice is body scan meditation. Start by lying down or sitting in a comfortable position and closing your eyes. Then, slowly scan your body from head to toe, paying attention to any sensations you feel. Again, if your mind starts to wander, simply bring it back to the sensations in your body.

There are many other types of mindfulness meditation practices, so explore until you find one that feels right for you. Remember, the goal is not to achieve perfection but simply to be present in the moment and let go of stress and anxiety.

The Benefits of Mindfulness Meditation

Mindfulness meditation can offer many benefits for your physical and mental health. Research has shown that mindfulness meditation can help reduce stress, anxiety, and depression while also improving sleep quality and overall well-being.

Mindfulness meditation can also help to improve focus and concentration while also reducing rumination and negative thinking. Additionally, mindfulness meditation has been shown to boost immune function and even help to reduce chronic pain.

If you're interested in trying mindfulness meditation, there are many resources available to help you get started. There are many books, websites, apps, and classes that can provide guidance on how to meditate. You may also want to consider seeking out a qualified mindfulness teacher or practitioner who can help you get started with a practice that's right for you.

The Different Types of Mindfulness Meditation

Mindfulness meditation can take many different forms, each with its own unique benefits.

1. Mindfulness of the breath: This type of mindfulness meditation involves focusing on the breath and noticing the sensations that come with each inhale and exhales This helps to anchor the mind in the present moment and can be a great way to calm down when feeling anxious or stressed.

2. Body scan: A body scan is a form of mindfulness meditation where you focus your attention on each part of your body, from head to toe. This can help you to become more aware of any tension you may be holding in your body and can also be a great way to relax before sleep.

3. Loving-kindness: Loving-kindness meditation involves directing feelings of care and compassion towards yourself and others. This can help to increase positive emotions and reduce stress and anxiety.

4. Visualization: Visualization is a form of mindfulness meditation where you focus on a calming image or scene. This can help to relax the mind and body, and may also be used as a tool to achieve specific goals

such as improving performance in a sport or increasing productivity at work.

5. Sound Meditation: Sound Meditation is a form of mindfulness meditation that uses sound waves to achieve relaxation. This may be done by listening to recorded sounds such as rain or thunder, or by attending a live sound bath session where gongs or singing bowls are played.

Mindfulness meditation can be a great way to reduce stress and anxiety, improve sleep, and increase focus and concentration. There are many different types of mindfulness meditation, so there is sure to be one that is right for you.

Pros and Cons of Mindfulness Meditation

Mindfulness meditation has become a popular way to reduce stress, improve focus, and promote overall well-being. But what is mindfulness meditation and what are the pros and cons of this type of practice?

Mindfulness meditation is a form of mindfulness that involves focusing your attention on the present moment. This can be done by paying attention to your breath, body, thoughts, and feelings. The goal of mindfulness meditation is to become more aware of your thoughts and feelings so that you can better control them.

There are many benefits of mindfulness meditation, including reducing stress, improving focus, and promoting overall well-being. However, there are also some potential drawbacks to this type of practice. Here are some pros and cons of mindfulness meditation:

Pros:

-Reduces stress

-Improves focus

-Promotes overall well-being

Cons:

-May not be suitable for everyone

-Can be difficult to stick with

Conclusion

Mindful meditation is a form of mindfulness that has been practised for centuries. It involves focusing your attention on the present moment and letting go of distractions. Mindfulness meditation has many benefits, including reducing stress, improving focus, and promoting overall well-being. However, it is not suitable for everyone and can be difficult to stick with. It can be used as a tool to help focus the mind, relax the body, and reduce stress. There are many benefits to mindful meditation, such as increased mental clarity and decreased anxiety. If you're looking to improve your well-being, consider giving mindful meditation a try.

Mindfulness meditation is not suitable for everyone and it can be difficult to stick with. If you're considering starting a mindfulness practice, it's important to consult with a qualified teacher or practitioner to ensure that it's right for you.

Mindfulness meditation can be a great way to improve your mental and physical well-being. However, it's important to understand the pros and cons of this type of practice before getting started.

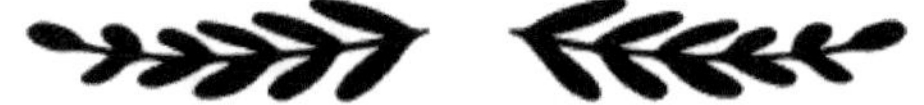

CHAPTER TWELVE

HOW TO DO DEEP BREATHING

DEEP BREATHING BRINGS thinking and shallow breathing brings shallow thinking. – Elsie Lincoln Benedict

You may have heard of deep breathing and how it can help with relaxation, but what is it and how do you do it correctly? Deep breathing is a type of slow, controlled breathing that allows you to take in more oxygen and expel more carbon dioxide. This helps to improve your overall respiratory function.

There are many benefits of deep breathing, including reducing stress, improving sleep quality, and reducing anxiety. Additionally, deep breathing can also help to improve your cardiovascular health. If you're looking to incorporate deep breathing into your daily routine, here are a few tips on how to do it correctly.

1. Sit or lie down in a comfortable position.

2. Place one hand on your stomach and the other on your chest.

3. Breathe in slowly through your nose, allowing your stomach to expand.

4. Breathe out slowly through your mouth.

5. Repeat this process for 10-15 minutes.

If you find it difficult to focus on your breath, try counting each inhale and exhale. You can also place one hand on your stomach and the other on your chest to make sure that you are breathing from your diaphragm. Remember, the goal is to breathe from your stomach and not your chest. Doing this correctly will help improve the quality of your deep breathing.

Deep breathing is an essential part of many relaxation and meditation techniques. It can also be used as a standalone tool to promote relaxation and reduce stress. There are a few different ways to do deep breathing, but the most important thing is to make sure that you're breathing from your diaphragm.

This means that your stomach should expand when you breathe in, rather than your chest. Here are a few tips on how to do deep breathing: 1. Sit or lie down in a comfortable position. 2. Place one hand on your stomach and the other on your chest. 3. Breathe in slowly through your nose, allowing your stomach to expand. 4. Breathe out slowly through your mouth. 5. Repeat this process for 10-15 minutes.

What is deep breathing?

When you breathe deeply, it means that you are taking in more oxygen and exhaling more carbon dioxide. This is because deep breathing allows your lungs to fully inflate and deflate, which increases the amount of oxygen that your body is able to take in. Deep breathing also helps to massage your internal organs, which can improve their function. Additionally, deep breathing has been shown to reduce stress and anxiety levels, as well as improve sleep quality.

Deep breathing is a simple, yet effective way to promote relaxation and reduce stress. It can be done anywhere, at any time, and requires no special equipment. The most important thing is to make sure that you're breathing from your diaphragm. This means that your stomach should expand when you breathe in, rather than your chest. Deep breathing is an effective way to relax because it slows down the heart rate and lowers blood pressure. When done correctly, deep breathing can also help to improve digestion and relieve tension headaches.

How to do deep breathing

When you are feeling stressed or anxious, one of the best things you can do is take some deep breaths. Deep breathing helps to oxygenate your blood, which can calm your body and mind. It is also a great way to get rid of any toxins that may be building up in your body.

To do deep breathing, start by finding a comfortable place to sit or lie down. Then, close your eyes and focus on your breath. Slowly inhale through your nose, filling up your stomach with air. Once your stomach is full, exhale slowly through your mouth. Repeat this process for 10-20 minutes.

If you find it difficult to focus on your breath, try counting each inhale and exhale. You can also place one hand on your stomach and the other on your chest to make sure that you are breathing from your diaphragm.

Deep breathing is a simple, yet effective way to promote relaxation and reduce stress. It can be done anywhere, at any time, and requires no special equipment. The most important thing is to make sure that you're breathing from your diaphragm. This means that your stomach should expand when you breathe in, rather than your chest. Deep breathing is an effective way to relax because it slows down the heart rate and lowers blood pressure. When done correctly, deep breathing can also help to improve digestion and relieve tension headaches.

The different types of deep breathing

There are many different types of deep breathing exercises, each with its own benefits.

One popular type of deep breathing is diaphragmatic breathing, also known as belly breathing. This type of breathing helps to massage the internal organs and improve circulation. It is also said to help with relaxation and stress relief.

Another popular type of deep breathing is alternate nostril breathing. This type of breathing is said to help clear the nasal passages and improve respiratory function. It is also said to help calm the mind and body, and promote balance in the nervous system.

Still another popular type of deep breathing is the four-fold breath, or square breath. This type of breath helps to increase lung capacity and improve the oxygenation of the blood. It is also said to help with relaxation and stress relief.

Finally, a type of deep breathing that is gaining popularity is Wim Hof Breathing. This type of breathing is said to help improve respiratory function, increase lung capacity, and promote a sense of calm. It is also said to help with cold exposure and boost the immune system.

The benefits of deep breathing

Deep breathing has many potential benefits, including:

improved circulation

massage of the internal organs

relaxation of the mind and body

improvement in respiratory function

increased lung capacity

improved oxygenation of the blood

boosting of the immune system.

When to do deep breathing

There are a few times when deep breathing can be especially helpful:

1. When you're feeling anxious or stressed

Deep breathing is a simple but effective way to calm the nervous system. It can help to control anxiety and manage stress.

2. When you're in pain

Deep breathing can help to ease both physical and emotional pain. It can also help to relax tense muscles.

3. When you need more energy

Deep breathing oxygenates the blood and gives the body an energy boost. If you're feeling tired, taking some deep breaths may help you to feel more alert and energized.

4. When you want to improve your sleep

Deep breathing can help to relax and prepare the body for sleep. If you have trouble falling asleep or staying asleep, deep breathing may help you to sleep better.

5. When you're pregnant

Deep breathing can help to ease stress and anxiety during pregnancy. It can also help to prepare the body for labour and delivery.

6. When you're sick

Deep breathing can help to clear congestion and make it easier to breathe when you're sick. It can also help to reduce fever and speed up the healing process.

7. When you're recovering from an injury

Deep breathing can help to reduce pain and swelling after an injury. It can also help to speed up the healing process.

8. When you want to improve your athletic performance

Deep breathing can help to improve stamina and endurance. It can also help to prevent pain and injuries during physical activity.

Conclusion

Deep breathing is a simple but powerful technique that can help to reduce stress and promote relaxation. By taking slow, deep breaths, you can ease both your mind and body. With regular practice, deep breathing can become second nature - something that you do automatically when you're feeling stressed or anxious. Give it a try the next time you're feeling overwhelmed or tense; you may be surprised at how quickly and effectively it works.

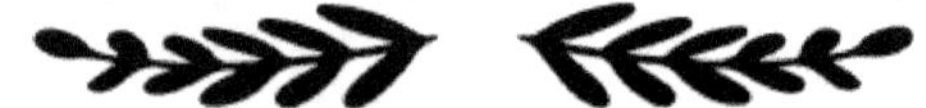

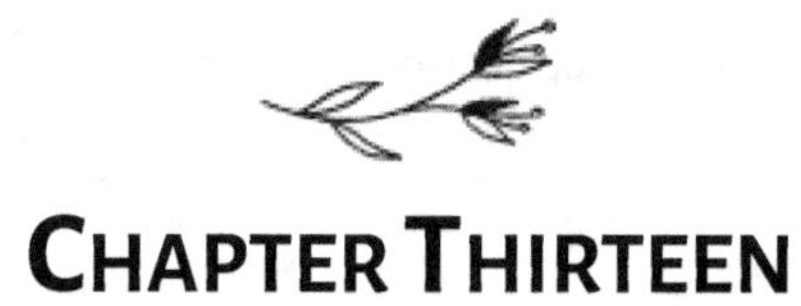

CHAPTER THIRTEEN

WHAT IS MUSIC THERAPY?

"LISTENING TO MUSIC HAS a positive impact on our health, by helping us recover faster when we experience stress, and through the reduction of the stress hormone cortisol, to help us achieve a calm state or homeostasis."

--Alex Doman, Music Producer and author of Healing at the Speed of Sound

Music therapy is the use of music to improve mental and physical health. It is a form of therapy that uses music to address the physical, emotional, mental, and social needs of individuals. Music therapy is an evidence-based practice that has been shown to be effective for a variety of populations, including those with mental health disorders, developmental disabilities, medical conditions, and more.

While research on the effectiveness of music therapy is still in its early stages, there is some evidence that it can be helpful for conditions like depression, anxiety, and chronic pain. Music therapy may also be beneficial for people who are dealing with trauma or substance abuse.

If you're curious about whether music therapy might be right for you, talk to your doctor or a licensed music therapist.

How does music therapy work?

Music therapy is the clinical and evidence-based use of music interventions to accomplish individualized goals within a therapeutic relationship. Music therapists use music safely and effectively to support clients' physical, emotional, cognitive, and social needs.

The best way to understand how music therapy works is to think about the different ways that music can be used therapeutically. Music can be used as a form of relaxation or stress relief, it can be used to help with focus and concentration, it can be used to promote movement and physical activity, and it can be used to express emotions.

Music therapists are trained to select music that is appropriate for each individual client and goal, and they will often use different techniques such as song writing, improvising, listening, or playing an instrument. The therapist will also create a safe and supportive environment where the client can feel comfortable exploring their feelings and thoughts through music.

There is a growing body of research that supports the effectiveness of music therapy. Music therapy has been shown to be effective for a variety of populations and issues, including anxiety, depression, pain management, stress relief, and more.

The benefits of music therapy

Music therapy is an effective form of treatment for a wide range of conditions and disorders. Some of the benefits of music therapy include:

The different types of music therapy

Music therapy is an evidence-based clinical use of music interventions to accomplish individualized goals within a therapeutic relationship.

Music therapists are trained in both music and counselling and must complete an accredited music therapy program to be credentialed. There are different types of music therapy that can be used to address a variety of needs, such as:

• Active music therapy: This type of therapy involves the client is actively involved in the music-making process, often through singing or playing an instrument.

• Receptive music therapy: This type of therapy involves the client listening to music, often with the help of headphones, and allowing the music to work its way into their subconscious.

• Analytical music therapy: This type of therapy uses musical elements such as rhythm, melody, and harmony to help people understand their emotions and thoughts.

• Improvisational music therapy: This type of therapy encourages clients to spontaneously create musical ideas in the moment, often with the help of a therapist who plays an accompanying instrument.

• Guided imagery and music (GIM): This type of therapy involves the client listening to music with the help of headphones while also imagining themselves in peaceful or happy settings.

The type of music therapy that is used will depend on the needs of the client. For example, someone who is struggling with anxiety may benefit from active music therapy, while someone who is dealing with depression may find receptive music therapy more helpful.

The benefits of music therapy

Music therapy has been shown to be an effective treatment for a variety of mental and physical health conditions. Some of the potential benefits of music therapy include:

• reducing stress and anxiety

• improving mood and sense of well-being

• aiding in pain management

• improving sleep quality

• increasing social interaction

• promoting motor skills development

• enhancing memory and cognitive functioning

How to find a music therapist

If you or a loved one is seeking music therapy services, there are a few things to keep in mind. First, it is important to find a board-certified music therapist (MT-BC). Board certification ensures that the music therapist has completed the necessary academic and clinical training to be considered an expert in the field.

There are a few ways to locate board-certified music therapists in your area. The American Music Therapy Association's (AMTA) website offers a searchable database of MT-BCs. You can also contact your local hospitals, hospices, nursing homes, and rehabilitation facilities to inquire about music therapy services.

Once you have located a few potential candidates, it is important to schedule an initial consultation. This will give you an opportunity to learn more about the therapist's qualifications and approach to treatment. It will also allow you to ask any questions you may have about music therapy.

During the consultation, be sure to ask about the therapist's experience working with clients who have similar needs as yourself or your loved one. It is also important to inquire about the type of music that will be used during therapy sessions and whether or not there are any risks involved.

After meeting with several different therapists, take some time to reflect on each individual before making a decision. Choose the therapist that you feel most comfortable with and who you believe will be best able to meet your needs or the needs of your loved one.

Music therapy is a relatively new field, but it has already helped countless individuals improve their quality of life. If you are looking for an alternative or supplemental treatment for yourself or a loved one, consider music therapy.

Conclusion

Music therapy is a type of therapy that uses music to help people with physical, emotional, or mental health issues. Music therapy can be used to help people relax, ease anxiety, and improve their mood. It can also be used to help people with more serious conditions like Alzheimer's disease, dementia, and ADHD.

If you're interested in music therapy, talk to your doctor or a licensed music therapist to see if it's right for you.

Music therapy is an effective form of treatment for a wide range of conditions and disorders. Some of the benefits of music therapy include: reducing anxiety and stress, enhancing memory and concentration, improving coordination and motor skills, promoting physical and emotional healing, and providing a sense of well-being.

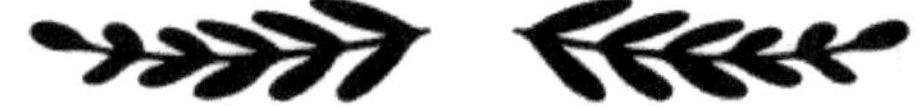

CHAPTER FOURTEEN

HOW TO TAKE CARE OF OUR MIND

"WHEN WE CARE FOR ourselves as our very own beloved—with naps, healthy food, clean sheets, a lovely cup of tea—we can begin to give in wildly generous ways to the world, from abundance. —Anne Lamott, author

We often think of taking care of our physical health as being the most important thing we can do for ourselves. However, our mental health is just as important, if not more so. In this blog post, we will explore how to take care of our mind. From getting enough sleep to exercise and more, read on to learn more about how you can keep your mind healthy and happy.

We all know that we should take care of our bodies by eating healthy foods and exercising regularly. However, we often forget that our mental health is just as important. In fact, our mental health can have a big impact on our physical health. That's why it's so important to find ways to keep our mind healthy and happy.

Here, we will explore how to take care of our mind. From getting enough sleep to exercise and more, read on to learn more about how you can keep your mind healthy and happy.

The mind-body connection

There is a lot of research that suggests that our physical and mental health are connected. For example, studies have shown that chronic stress can lead to physical health problems like heart disease, Alzheimer's disease, and obesity. Conversely, physical illness can lead to mental health problems like anxiety and depression.

It's important to take care of both our physical and mental health, as they are both interconnected. Here are some tips on how to take care of our mind:

1. Get enough sleep: Sleep is important for both our physical and mental health. It helps our bodies repair and regenerate, and it also helps improve our mood, memory, and cognitive function. Most adults need 7-8 hours of sleep per night.

2. Eat healthy: Eating a healthy diet can help improve our mood, memory, focus, and energy levels. Include plenty of fruits, vegetables, whole grains, lean proteins, and healthy fats in your diet. Avoid processed foods, sugary drinks, and excessive amounts of caffeine.

3. Exercise regularly: Exercise releases chemicals in the brain that help improve mood and reduce stress levels. It also helps improve sleep quality and increase energy levels. aim for at least 30 minutes of moderate-intensity exercise most days of the week.

4. Take breaks during the day: When we're feeling overwhelmed or stressed out, it's important to take a break from whatever is causing us stress. Take a few deep breaths, go for a walk, or just step away from the situation for a few minutes.

5. Connect with others: Spending time with family and friends can help reduce stress levels and improve mood. Whether you're catching up over the phone, meeting up for coffee, or spending time together in person, social interaction is important for our mental health.

6. Do something you enjoy: Doing things we enjoy can help reduce stress and improve our mood. Make time for hobbies, interests, and activities that make you happy.

7. Practice relaxation techniques: Relaxation techniques like yoga, meditation, and deep breathing can help reduce stress levels and improve our overall well-being.

8. Seek professional help: If you're struggling with anxiety, depression, or any other mental health issue, it's important to seek professional help. A therapist can help you identify and manage stressors in your life, as well as provide tools and resources for coping with mental health issues.

The benefits of taking care of our mind

When it comes to taking care of our mind, there are many benefits to doing so. For one, it can help reduce stress and anxiety levels. Additionally, it can improve our mood and cognitive function. Finally, taking care of our mind can also lead to better sleep and overall physical health.

One of the most important benefits of taking care of our mind is that it can help reduce stress and anxiety levels. Stress and anxiety can have a negative impact on our mental and physical health. Therefore, by reducing these levels, we can improve our overall well-being. Additionally, taking care of our mind can also improve our mood.

Mood swings can be caused by a variety of factors, including stress and anxiety. Therefore, by improving our mood, we can reduce the likelihood of experiencing mood swings. Finally, taking care of our mind can also lead to better sleep. Poor sleep can have a negative impact on our physical and mental health. Therefore, by improving our sleep habits, we can improve our overall health.

The different ways to take care of our mind

There are many different ways that we can take care of our mind. We can meditate, do yoga, or even just take a few moments to breathe deeply and relax.

We can also read uplifting books, listen to calming music, or spend time in nature. Anything that helps us to relax and feel good can be beneficial for our mind.

It's important to find what works for us and to make sure that we make time for self-care. It can be easy to get caught up in the hustle and bustle of everyday life and forget to take care of ourselves. But if we don't make time for ourselves, we can end up feeling stressed out and overwhelmed.

So take some time for yourself each day, even if it's just a few minutes. Breathe deeply, relax, and enjoy the moment. It's your chance to recharge and refocus so that you can face the world with a clear mind.

1. Meditation

One of the best ways to take care of our mind is through meditation. Meditation helps us to focus and connect with our inner thoughts and feelings. It can be a very powerful tool in reducing stress and anxiety.

There are many different types of meditation, so it's important to find one that works for you. You can meditate on your own or with a group. There are also guided meditation programs available online or through apps.

2. Yoga

Yoga is another great way to take care of our minds. Yoga helps to improve our flexibility, strength, and balance. It also helps to calm our minds and relax our bodies.

There are many different types of yoga, so it's important to find one that works for you. You can do yoga at home or take a class at a studio. There are also online classes available if you prefer to do yoga in the comfort of your own home.

3. Breathing Exercises

Breathing exercises are another simple but effective way to take care of our minds. They help us to focus and relax our bodies by increasing the oxygen flow to our brains.

There are many different types of breathing exercises, so it's important to find ones that work for you. You can do them anywhere and at any time.

4. Relaxation Techniques

Relaxation techniques are another great way to take care of our minds. They help us to focus and relax our bodies by releasing tension.

There are many different types of relaxation techniques, so it's important to find ones that work for you. You can do them anywhere and at any time.

5. Mindfulness

Mindfulness is a practice that helps us to be present in the moment and aware of our thoughts and feelings. It can be very helpful in reducing stress and anxiety.

There are many different ways to be mindful, so it's important to find what works for you. You can practice mindfulness on your own or with a group. There are also online programs available if you prefer to do mindfulness in the comfort of your own home.

6. Journaling

Journaling is a great way to take care of our minds. It helps us to process our thoughts and feelings and can be very therapeutic.

There are many different ways to journal, so it's important to find what works for you. You can journal in a notebook or on your computer. There are also online journals available if you prefer to journal in the comfort of your own home.

7. Art Therapy

Art therapy is another great way to take care of our minds. It helps us to express our thoughts and feelings in a creative way.

There are many different types of art therapy, so it's important to find what works for you. You can do art therapy on your own or with a group. There are also online classes available if you prefer to do art therapy in the comfort of your own home.

8. Nature

Nature is a great way to take care of our minds. It helps us to connect with the world around us and can be very soothing.

There are many different ways to connect with nature, so it's important to find what works for you. You can go for a walk in the park or spend time in your backyard. You can also visit a nearby lake or forest.

9. Exercise

Exercise is another great way to take care of our minds. It helps to release endorphins which have mood-boosting effects. Exercise also helps to improve our sleep and reduces stress and anxiety.

There are many different types of exercise, so it's important to find what works for you. You can do aerobic exercise, such as walking or running. You can also do strength-training exercises, such as weightlifting. There are also many different types of yoga and Pilates available if you prefer a gentler form of exercise.

10. Connect with Others

Connecting with others is another great way to take care of our minds. It helps us to feel supported and loved. We can connect with others through family, friends, or even online communities.

It's important to find what works for you and to make sure that you are connecting with people who make you feel good. If you are feeling isolated or lonely, reach out to someone and make a connection today.

11. Get Enough Sleep

Getting enough sleep is crucial for our minds and body. It helps us to feel rested and rejuvenated. It also helps to reduce stress and anxiety.

There are many different ways to get a good night's sleep, so it's important to find what works for you. You can create a bedtime routine, such as reading or taking a bath before bed. You can also make sure that your sleeping environment is dark, quiet, and cool.

12. Eat Healthily

Eating healthy is another great way to take care of our minds. Eating nutritious foods helps our body to function at its best. It also helps to reduce stress and anxiety.

There are many different ways to eat healthy, so it's important to find what works for you. You can eat a variety of fruits, vegetables, and whole grains. You can also make sure to include lean protein and healthy fats in your diet.

13. Reduce Stress

Reducing stress is one of the best things we can do for our mind and body. Stress can have harmful effects on our health, so it's important to find ways to reduce it in our lives.

There are many different ways to reduce stress, so it's important to find what works for you. You can do relaxation techniques, such as yoga or meditation. You can also make sure to get enough sleep and exercise.

14. Seek Help

If you are struggling to take care of your mind, it's important to seek
help. There are many resources available to help you if you are struggling
with mental health issues.

15. Identify your stressors

What are the things in your life that tend to cause you to stress? Once
you know what your triggers are, you can start to work on finding ways
to eliminate or reduce them.

Conclusion

It's important to take care of our minds just as much as we take care of
our bodies. We can do this by meditating, practising mindfulness, and
spending time in nature. Taking care of our minds will help reduce stress,
improve our mood, and promote overall well-being.

We all know that we should take care of our bodies by eating healthy
foods and exercising regularly. However, we often forget that our mental
health is just as important. In fact, our mental health can have a big

impact on our physical health. That's why it's so important to find ways to keep our minds healthy and happy.

Here, we will explore how to take care of our minds. From getting enough sleep to exercise and more, read on to learn more about how you can keep your mind healthy and happy.

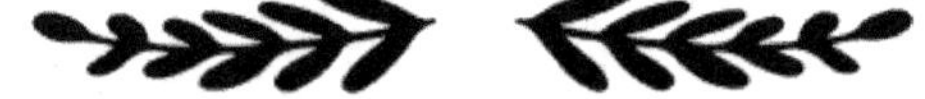

CHAPTER FIFTEEN

FULL BOOK SUMMARY OF "MIND YOUR MIND"

CHAPTER 1-**DEVELOP DAILY SELF CARE Mental Habits**

Self-care is crucial for maintaining good mental health. By developing daily self-care habits, you can take charge of your mental health and well-being. These habits will help you to cope with stress, deal with difficult emotions, and make better decisions for your overall health and happiness.

Chapter 2-**Develop intellectual well being**

Intellectual well-being is a state of being in which a person's intellectual needs are met and they are able to think critically and creatively. A person with intellectual well-being is curious and open-minded and has a growth mindset. They are also able to manage their emotions, set and achieve goals, and deal with stress in healthy ways.

There are many different ways to develop intellectual well-being. Certain things, however, are more significant than others. Reading, writing, being curious, challenging yourself, and taking care of your body are all great ways to improve your intellectual well-being.

There is no one-size-fits-all answer to the question of how to develop intellectual well-being. However, there are some key things that you can do to help yourself in this regard. Firstly, make sure that you engage in activities that challenge your mind on a regular basis. This could involve anything from reading complex books to working on difficult puzzles. Secondly, try to surround yourself with people who are stimulating and intellectually curious, as this will encourage you to think more deeply about the world around you. Finally, don't be afraid to ask questions and seek out new information; the more you know, the easier it will be to develop a well-rounded understanding of the world and everything in i t.

Intellectual wellness is important for both an individual and society. That said, there are many ways to improve it. One of the most important things is to regularly read, write, be curious, challenge yourself, and take care of your body. Spending time with people who challenge your thinking and help you grow intellectually is also important. By following these tips and optimizing your actions, you can cultivate a rich inner life that will lead to a fulfilling existence.

Chapter 3-**Improve mental health**

If you're looking for ways to improve your mental health, there are a number of things you can do. From getting regular exercise and making sure you're getting enough sleep, to eating a healthy diet and spending time with supportive people, there are many small steps you can take that will make a big difference. Remember, it's important to be kind to yourself – give yourself time and space to heal, and don't hesitate to ask for help when you need it.

Chapter 4-**How to practice mindfulness**

Mindfulness meditation is a form of mindfulness that can be practised anywhere, at any time. All you need is a comfortable place to sit or recline, and the willingness to focus your attention on your breath and the present moment. With regular practice, mindfulness meditation can help you learn how to better control your thoughts and emotions, and improve your overall well-being.

If you're interested in mindfulness but aren't quite sure how to get started, there are many resources available to help you, including books, apps, and online courses. The important thing is to find a way that works for you and that you can stick with. Mindfulness takes practice, so be patient with yourself and keep at it!

Mindfulness is a state of being present in the moment, without judgment. It's an awareness that comes from paying attention to your thoughts, emotions, and sensations in the present moment.

When you're mindful, you're not trying to change anything or achieve anything. You're simply observing and accepting what is. This can be a difficult concept to grasp, but with practice, it can be very liberating.

There are many benefits to practising mindfulness, including reducing stress, improving focus and concentration, promoting a sense of well-being, and more. If you're interested in incorporating mindfulness into your life, there are many ways to do so, including formal mindfulness meditation, body scan mindfulness, walking mindfulness, and eating mindfulness.

The important thing is to find a way that works for you and that you can stick with. Mindfulness takes practice, so be patient with yourself and keep at it!

Mindfulness can be a difficult concept to grasp, but with practice, it can be very liberating.

There are many benefits to practising mindfulness, including reducing stress, improving focus and concentration, promoting a sense of well-being, and more.

Chapter 5-**Improve focus and concentration**

There are a number of ways to improve focus and concentration, and it really depends on what works best for you. Some people find that listening to music or white noise helps them to focus, while others prefer complete silence. Some people like to work in short bursts with frequent breaks, while others can maintain their focus for hours at a time. Experiment with different techniques and find what works best for you. And remember, even if you can't always maintain perfect focus, don't be too hard on yourself - we all have our off days!

Chapter 6-**Best relaxation techniques**

There is no one-size-fits-all answer to this question, as the best relaxation technique for you may vary depending on your individual needs and preferences. However, there are a few key things to keep in mind when choosing a relaxation technique that will help you find the one that works best for you.

First, consider what you want to achieve through relaxation. Do you want to reduce stress, improve sleep, or boost your mood? Once you know what your goal is, you can narrow down your options and choose a technique that is best suited to help you achieve it.

Second, think about what type of environment you feel most relaxed in. Do you prefer being outdoors in nature, or indoors in a quiet room? This will help guide you towards techniques that will be most effective for you.

Finally, consider your personal preferences and needs when choosing a relaxation technique. For example, if you have trouble sitting still, then a moving meditation like Tai Chi or Yoga might be a better option for you than something like mindfulness meditation. Trust your instincts and go with what feels right for you.

Chapter 7-**Boost your mood**

There are many ways to boost your mood, and it ultimately comes down to finding what works best for you. Experiment with different activities and strategies until you find a combination that works for you. And don't forget to give yourself some grace - sometimes feeling down is just a part of life. But by using these tips, you can hopefully increase the frequency of those good days.

Chapter 8-**Have a positive mindset**

Having a positive mindset is one of the most important things you can do for yourself. It's not always easy, but it's worth it. When you have a positive outlook on life, you're more likely to be successful, happy, and healthy. Here are a few tips to help you develop and maintain a positive mindset: 1. Be grateful for what you have. 2. Focus on the good in every situation. 3. Find humour in everyday situations. 4. Surround yourself with positive people. 5. Practice positive visualization. 6. Don't sweat the small stuff. 7. Take care of yourself physically and emotionally. 8. Be patient with yourself.

If you're looking to improve your life in any way, developing a positive mindset is a great place to start.

Chapter 9-**How to Identify Your Triggers**

Now that you know what a trigger is and how to identify your own, you can start to work on managing them. This may involve avoiding certain triggers altogether, or learning how to deal with them in a healthy way. If you're not sure where to start, talk to your doctor or a qualified mental health professional. They can help you develop a plan for dealing with your triggers and help you get on the road to recovery.

Chapter 10-**What is mindful meditation?**

Mindful meditation is a form of mindfulness that has been practised for centuries. It involves focusing your attention on the present moment and letting go of distractions. Mindfulness meditation has many benefits, including reducing stress, improving focus, and promoting overall well-being. However, it is not suitable for everyone and can be difficult to stick with. It can be used as a tool to help focus the mind, relax the body, and reduce stress. There are many benefits to mindful meditation, such as increased mental clarity and decreased anxiety. If you're looking to improve your well-being, consider giving mindful meditation a try.

Mindfulness meditation is not suitable for everyone and it can be difficult to stick with. If you're considering starting a mindfulness practice, it's important to consult with a qualified teacher or practitioner to ensure that it's right for you.

Mindfulness meditation can be a great way to improve your mental and physical well-being. However, it's important to understand the pros and cons of this type of practice before getting started.

Chapter 11-**How to do deep breathing**

Deep breathing is a simple but powerful technique that can help to reduce stress and promote relaxation. By taking slow, deep breaths, you can ease both your mind and body. With regular practice, deep breathing can become second nature - something that you do automatically when you're feeling stressed or anxious. Give it a try the next time you're feeling overwhelmed or tense; you may be surprised at how quickly and effectively it works.

Chapter 12-**What is music therapy?**

Music therapy is a type of therapy that uses music to help people with physical, emotional, or mental health issues. Music therapy can be used to help people relax, ease anxiety, and improve their mood. It can also be used to help people with more serious conditions like Alzheimer's disease, dementia, and ADHD.

If you're interested in music therapy, talk to your doctor or a licensed music therapist to see if it's right for you.

Music therapy is an effective form of treatment for a wide range of conditions and disorders. Some of the benefits of music therapy include: reducing anxiety and stress, enhancing memory and concentration, improving coordination and motor skills, promoting physical and emotional healing, and providing a sense of well-being.

Chapter 13-**How to take care of our mind**

It's important to take care of our minds just as much as we take care of our bodies. We can do this by meditating, practising mindfulness, and spending time in nature. Taking care of our minds will help reduce stress, improve our mood, and promote overall well-being.

We all know that we should take care of our bodies by eating healthy foods and exercising regularly. However, we often forget that our mental health is just as important. In fact, our mental health can have a big impact on our physical health. That's why it's so important to find ways to keep our minds healthy and happy.

Here, we will explore how to take care of our minds. From getting enough sleep to exercise and more, read on to learn more about how you can keep your mind healthy and happy.

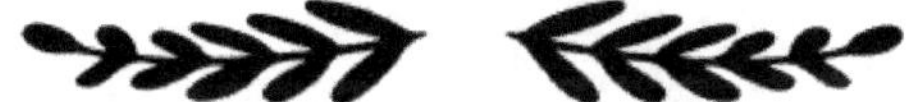

BEFORE YOU GO

P LEASE, SPARE A MINUTE to rate this book using the star ratings from 1-to-5, that usually pops up at the end of this publication. I appreciate your honest feedback, positive or negative. And if you have an extra moment to spare, could you rate the book on Amazon.

Thank you, and best regards.

Manjul

Special Note:

As most e book readers (including the Amazon Kindle) do not have a great internet browser interface, you might prefer to scan the QR Code below using your smart phone.

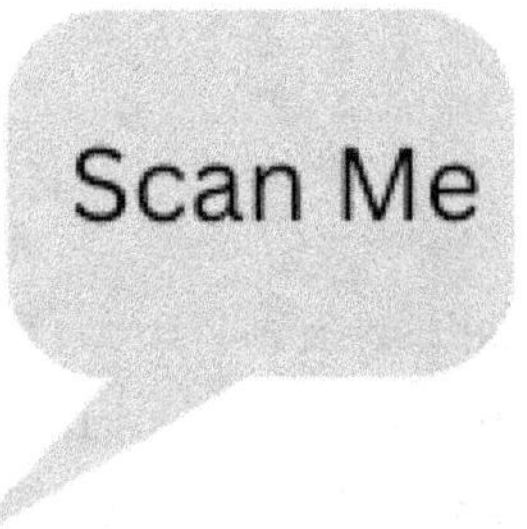

Scan this QR Code with your Smart Phone and leave a review

REFERENCES

1. Oliver Elbs 2005, *Neuro-Esthetics: Mapological foundations and applications (Map 2003)*, Munich.

2. ^ Jump up to:*a b c d* *"Mind". Encyclopedia Britannica. Archived from the original on 9 May 2021. Retrieved 31 May 2021.*

3. ^ *"mind". American Heritage Dictionary of the English Language. Houghton Mifflin Harcourt. 2016. Archived from the original on 2021-06-29. Retrieved 2021-06-29.*

4. ^ *"mind". Collins English Dictionary. HarperCollins. 2014. Archived from the original on 2021-06-29. Retrieved 2021-06-29.*

5. ^ Jump up to:*a b* *Clark, Andy (2014). Mindware. New*

York: Oxford University Press. pp. 14, 254–56. ISBN 978-0-19-982815-9.

6. ^ Smart, J.J.C., "The Mind/Brain Identity Theory Archived 2013-12-02 at the Wayback Machine", The Stanford Encyclopedia of Philosophy (Fall 2011 ed.), Edward N. Zalta (ed.)

7. ^ *"What is mind-brain identity theory?". SearchCIO. Tech target. WhatIs. Archived from the original on 2020-04-22. Retrieved 2020-05-26.*

8. ^ *Klopf, Harry (June 1975). "A comparison of natural and artificial intelligence". SIGART Bulletin. ACM (52): 11–13. doi :10.1145/1045236.1045237. S2CID 17852070.*

9. ^ Jump up to:[a] [b] [c] [d] *Karunamuni, N; Weerasekera, R (Jun 2017). "Theoretical Foundations to Guide Mindfulness Meditation: A Path to Wisdom". Current Psychology (submitted manuscript). **38** (3): 627–46. doi:10.1007/s12144-017-9631-7. S2CID 149024504. Archived from the original on 2019-10-24. Retrieved 2018-09-11.*

10. ^ Jump up to:[a] [b] [c] [d] *Karunamuni, N.D. (May 2015). "The Five-Aggregate Model of the Mind". SAGE Open. **5** (2). doi:10 .1177/2158244015583860.*

BOOKS BY THE SAME AUTHOR

BOOKS BY THE SAME AUTHOR

5 — The Innovative Mindset

https://www.amazon.com/Innovativ
e-Mindset-Innovation-Creativity-
Innovators-ebook/dp/B0CJ98N8M2

6 — The Eloquent Mindset

https://www.amazon.com/dp/
B0CM3D3VW1

7 — The Clear Mindset

https://www.amazon.com/dp
/B0CSSQ3MC6/

8 — The Positive
Thinking Mindset

https://www.amazon.com/dp
/B0CSSQ3MC6/

ABOUT THE AUTHOR

MANJUL TEWARI, A BLOGGER, best-selling author, and versatile writer, is the creative force behind the captivating 'Mindset Mastery Series' available on Amazon.

With an engaging and informative style, Manjul's writings transcend conventional boundaries, enriching the lives of readers worldwide. Delve deeper into Manjul's literary world and discover the transformational power of effective communication and mindset mastery.

Visit the **author's profile on Amazon** to explore the full range of captivating works. Uncover the magic of communication and mindset mastery through the lens of Manjul Tewari's literary adventure.